How *to* GROW & EAT *Your* OWN SUPER FOODS

BECKY DICKINSON

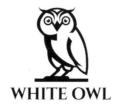

WHITE OWL

First published in Great Britain in 2018 by
PEN & SWORD WHITE OWL
An imprint of Pen & Sword Books Limited
47 Church Street
Barnsley
South Yorkshire
S70 2AS

ISBN 9781526714336

Printed and bound by Replika Press Pvt. Ltd

Design by Paul Wilkinson

Pen & Sword Books Limited incorporates the imprints of Atlas,
Archaeology, Aviation, Discovery, Family History, Fiction, History, Maritime, Military, Military
Classics, Politics, Select, Transport, True Crime, Air World, Frontline Publishing, Leo Cooper,
Remember When, Seaforth Publishing,
The Praetorian Press, Wharncliffe Local History, Wharncliffe Transport,
Wharncliffe True Crime and White Owl.

For a complete list of Pen & Sword titles please contact
PEN & SWORD BOOKS LIMITED
47 Church Street, Barnsley, South Yorkshire, S70 2AS, United Kingdom
E-mail: enquiries@pen-and-sword.co.uk
Website: www.pen-and-sword.co.uk

Or
PEN AND SWORD BOOKS
1950 Lawrence Rd, Havertown, PA 19083, USA
E-mail: Uspen-and-sword@casematepublishers.com
Website: www.penandswordbooks.com

Contents

Introduction

Super Soil

Part Two: Fruit and Veg ♥ Love ❋ Grow ☙ Eat

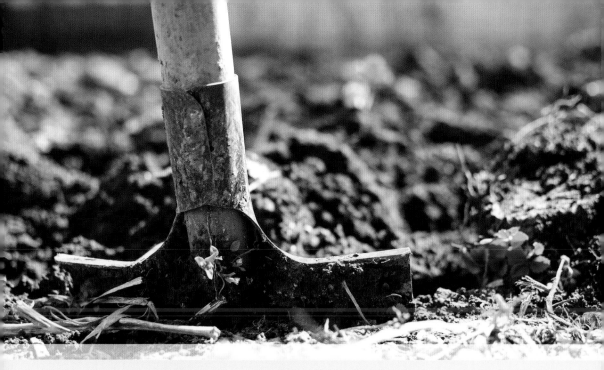

Introduction

FEW THINGS IN LIFE are quite as satisfying as growing your own food. There is something almost miraculous about scattering a few dry looking seeds over soil, then waking up a couple of weeks later, to a row of tiny green shoots.

As leaves unfurl and flowers give way to fruit, there is a simple yet profound pleasure in witnessing a seed's journey from plot to plate. Gardening is where science meets art, where nature meets nurture and where food and health unite.

Not only are home-grown fruits and vegetables infinitely sweeter, crunchier and more flavoursome than their shop-bought counterparts, they are also richer in vitamins, minerals and antioxidants, which are all at their peak when first picked. Yet we live in an age where 'superfoods' are marketed alongside convenience. We are urged to buy produce that will optimise our health without compromising our busy lifestyles; pre-packaged, ready prepared and unceasingly, unseasonably available.

Social media, magazines and the internet are awash with miracle diets, celebrity eating regimes and an ever-growing list of so-called superfoods that will help us live longer, healthier, happier lives. Yet often these foods have travelled miles across the globe and are tainted with chemicals that have been linked to the very diseases we hope to prevent. That bag of wilting kale has been sitting in a supermarket since Wednesday, that expensive punnet of blueberries was flown thousands of miles across the sea, those non-organic beetroot sweating beneath a layer of cling film may contain pesticide residues or heavy metals.

Fruits and vegetables, whether or not they fall into the superfood subset, are a vital part of our diet and an essential source of vitamins, minerals, antioxidants, fibre and other nutrients. But the best way to ensure you are getting the maximum benefit, and no nasty extras, from your greens (and reds and oranges and purples) is to sow and pick your own. The real super foods are the ones you have grown yourself and picked in season.

Growing your own produce is better for your health, better for the environment, and surprisingly easy to accomplish. You may not be able to grow strawberries in January, or watermelons in Scotland, but you can almost certainly grow at least some of what you eat. Few people have the time or space to become completely self-sufficient but it's amazing how much can be grown with minimal expertise and resources.

Whether you have an allotment the size of a leisure centre, a garden the size of a paddling pool, or just a medley of pots, growing even a little of the food you consume will enrich your health and life in myriad ways. It doesn't matter if you have never grown so much as a handful of cress seeds before, it's never too late, or too difficult, to pick up a trowel and learn on the job.

This book is not about eliminating every non-organic molecule from your daily existence, or obsessing about every grain of sugar. It's about the realistic, enjoyable and life-enhancing possibilities that can arise from a patch of soil – while still leaving room for cake and wine.

It's about taking control of some of what you eat and growing your way to better health through the fruits and vegetables of your own labour. Because gardening, especially edible gardening, is addictive for all the right reasons.

Super reasons to grow your own

People are gardeners for all sorts of reasons; pleasure, pride, necessity, food, financial reasons, environmental reasons, physical exercise, fresh air and escapism – nothing helps assuage the stresses and anxieties of everyday life quite like a couple of hours digging and weeding. For most people, it becomes a mixture of all of these things.

Growing your own produce is better for your health, better for the environment, and surprisingly easy to accomplish ...

Not only are conventionally-grown, mass-produced fruit and vegetables lacking in taste, they are also lacking in nutritional quality ...

The more you get into gardening, the more you discover you can't live without it. There is an intense satisfaction in witnessing all that sweat, mud and backache blossom into a magnificent abundance of flowers, fruits and vegetables. And there is overwhelming evidence that being immersed in nature is hugely beneficial for our physical and mental wellbeing.

I started growing things when I was around eight years old, when I stuck a lemon pip into a yoghurt pot filled with earth and hid it in the airing cupboard to see what would happen. It grew! And the seeds of addiction were sown.

I grew stuff anywhere and everywhere; window boxes in London, back yards in Wales, tiny, dank gardens in the suburbs, even the back of my car (cars make brilliant greenhouses) until I finally landed an allotment and threw myself into it with naive gusto. Fortunately, there were plenty of people with decades more experience than I had, who could steer me in the right direction when needed.

But it wasn't until children came along that I really began growing for health. Instinctively, I felt that there was something unsavoury about shop-bought fruit and veg: watery carrots, insipid salad, waxy apples, spongy aubergines, homogenous courgettes. No wonder so many children refused to eat vegetables. But flavour is only half the story. Not only are conventionally-grown, mass-produced fruit and vegetables lacking in taste, they are also lacking in nutritional quality.

Ground-breaking research carried out at Newcastle University found significant nutritional differences between organic and non-organic crops, with organic ones containing substantially more antioxidants.[1] Concentrations of key antioxidants such as polyphenolics, which have been linked to a reduced risk of chronic diseases, including cardiovascular and neurodegenerative diseases and certain cancers, were found to be up to 60 per cent higher in organically-grown crops.

In fact, it was discovered that switching to eating organic fruit, vegetable and cereals – and food made from them – would provide additional antioxidants equivalent to eating between 1-2 extra portions of fruit and vegetables a day. The study, which was published in the *British Journal of Nutrition*, also found that organic crops were far less likely to be contaminated with pesticides and toxic heavy metals such as cadmium, which is one of only three metal contaminants along with lead and mercury for which the European Commission has set maximum permitted contamination levels in food. Cadmium, which is

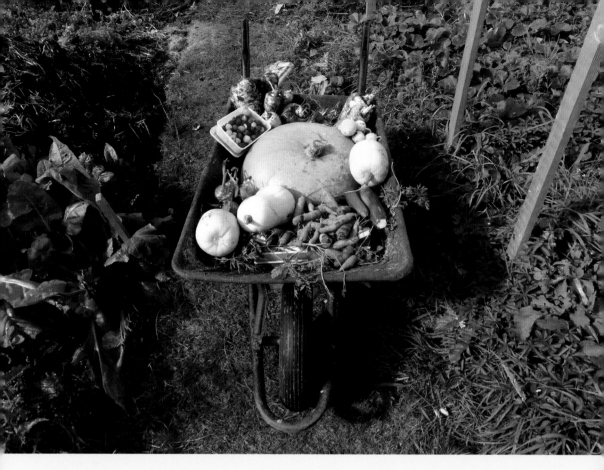

classified as a human carcinogen, was found to be almost 50 per cent lower in organic crops, along with pesticide residues, which were four times more likely to be found in conventionally-grown crops.

Harvesting your own healthy crops is the final reward for all that effort.

More than 300 chemicals such as benzalkonium chloride and thiophanate-methyl can be used in non-organic farming and these may still be present in non-organic food, even after washing and cooking. Government reports reveal that pesticide residues are found in a high percentage of UK foods, and many fruits and vegetables contain traces of not just one, but several different chemicals.[2] For example, routine testing of blueberries and blackberries in 2015, found that 55 out of 96 samples contained pesticide residues, four of which measured above maximum residue levels, and 38 samples contained multiple residues – in some cases as many as six different chemicals.[3] In short, organically grown fruit and vegetables are higher in healthy substances, and lower in potentially harmful ones. They also taste better.

But shop-bought organic foods are often prohibitively expensive. Throw in the word superfood, and you can double, or even triple, your shopping bill. The obvious, affordable and entirely feasible

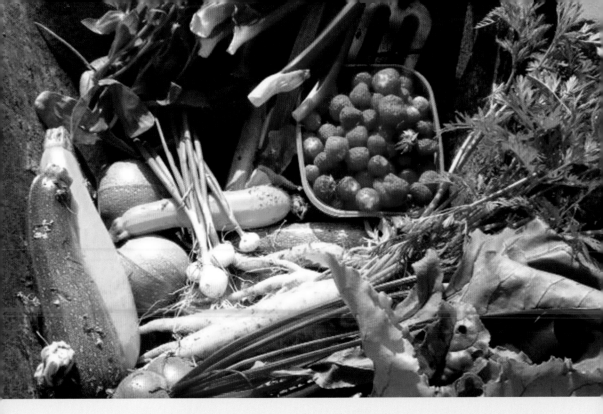

solution is to grow it yourself. Growing your own food means super quality at a fraction of the cost.

Of course, there will be challenges along the way: battalions of slugs; outbursts of weather; seedlings that fail to get off the ground (literally;) and people who tell you it's not worth the hassle. Ignore them. Because in the end, nature prevails and you will discover that you don't need to be an expert to grow enough food to eat, or to feed a family. What's more, you can feel secure in the knowledge that the food you grow is nourishing, fresh and safe and is in fact, a super food. And nothing beats the satisfaction of that.

Superfoods: fad or fact?

There was a time when all vegetables were grown on a level playing field, or at least an even patch of roughly-cultivated soil. Cabbages, parsnips, carrots, beans and cauliflower shared equal status on the vegetable plot and in the supermarket. There was no such thing as a vegetable hierarchy, although asparagus was regarded as somewhat posh, owing to its price tag and short season of availability. And while Popeye was famous for his (tinned) spinach-powered biceps, even that had yet to be described as a superfood. Kale on the other hand was noted for being slightly tough and bitter; beetroot usually came out of jars and tasted predominantly of vinegar, and few people outside of Asia had heard of goji berries.

Fast forward a few years, and these previously maligned or unfamiliar crops are enjoying a surge in popularity, thanks to their reinvention as superfoods, a title which has been bestowed upon foods said to have special health benefits.

The term quickly became a buzzword, leading to the creation of a kind of super league of health foods, with more and more products joining the club; blueberries, quinoa, chia, pomegranate, acai, coconut water, wheatgrass, spirulina, and a whole collection of suddenly sought-after and often exotic plants and berries.

The only thing these otherwise unrelated crops had in common was their alleged ability to protect us from aging and disease, usually due to their high concentration of antioxidants – the compounds that mop up free-radicals, the unstable molecules that can harm our DNA, leading to the development of diseases and disorders. Yet wrapping fruits and vegetables in scientific jargon and extravagant health claims only separates us from their natural, uncomplicated appeal, just as pulverizing a pile of leafy veg into a medicinal-looking green juice turns intrinsic healthy goodness into something that must be endured, rather than enjoyed.

There is no denying that so-called superfoods are generally healthy in their own right and can have a positive function in a balanced diet, but it is also fair to say that the main beneficiaries are the large-scale producers and companies who sell them.

Nutritionists are often dismissive about the term superfood and spokesperson for the British Dietetic Association, Michelle McGuinness, says it should be treated with healthy scepticism.

'When foods are marketed as "superfoods" the public generally have the perception that this food is healthy and often more superior than other similar foods, it gives it a "health halo". This leaves health conscious members of the public believing that they have made the healthiest choice, often without understanding why, regardless of whether it is or not. The foods are sometimes marketed as "super" off the back of a scientific study which may not be robust or good quality, may not be done on humans or may be based on high concentration doses of nutrients which may not be palatable or achievable when you look at how much of the nutrient content is in the "superfood". Given that the benefit of the "superfood" is very rarely clear to the consumer, and that the term itself is rather vague, the main objective is

There is no denying that so-called superfoods are generally healthy in their own right ...

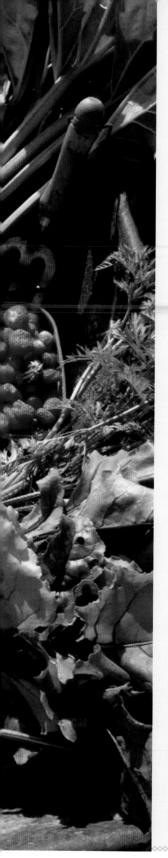

generally to appeal to the health food market, raise the sales of a product or to be in keeping with latest food trend.'

Although the word superfood is widely used, it has no regulatory approval and is not a legally recognised term. In fact, the European Union has banned the marketing of products as 'superfoods', unless backed up by a specific authorised health claim that explains to consumers why the product is good for their health.[4]

This is not to say that foods popularly known as superfoods aren't good for you. Of course they are, but no one food can cure cancer, prevent diabetes or reverse Alzheimer's disease. A balanced, healthy diet involves eating a wide variety of foods, not simply swallowing the hype. Often, alternative fruits and vegetables will provide similar benefits without the price tag. Blackberries, for example, are rich in antioxidants and contain more than double the vitamin C of blueberries – and are freely available in season. Broccoli is not only cheaper than kale, but contains many of the same vital nutrients including vitamins C and K, calcium, folate and beta-carotene. And raspberries contain similar amounts of fibre to goji berries, but with far less sugar.

The danger is that by focusing on a handful of costly, often exotic, 'superfoods', we ignore the plethora of plants sitting on our doorstep and overlook their own super qualities. The humble cabbage, the ordinary carrot, the modest bean, the everyday onion, the essential garlic; they may not have had the benefit of a healthy marketing campaign or celebrity endorsement, but all can play a role in a super diet.

It's time to move away from 'superfoods' and focus instead on super foods – the home-grown, organically produced crops that are bursting with super properties.

This book will explore the nutritional benefits of a whole army of fruits and vegetables, not just the ones that make the headlines, and reveal how you can grow them yourself. There should be nothing mysterious, or clinical, or fashionable about growing super foods. People have been doing it for centuries and it's not rocket science (unless you're growing rocket that is, but even then, it's still not science.) The science is already contained within the seed, all you have to do is plant it, nurture it and enjoy it.

Not only will your home-grown produce taste better, it will also do you far more good than the chemically grown, supermarket-shelved imitations. In fact, any food can be a super food if you have grown it yourself.

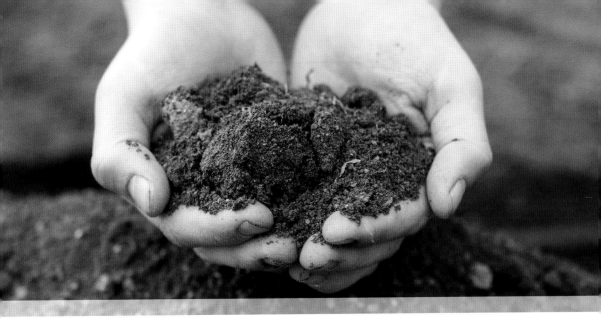

Super Soil

THE KEY TO GROWING super foods is to provide them with super soil. And the key to super soil is to nourish it with organic material like compost and manure, and not to bombard it with artificial fertilisers, pesticides, weed killers and fungicides. It may look brown and uninspiring, but the mud beneath your feet, is just as important as the food you grow in it.

Of course, even kale sown in a nutrient-depleted, chemically-laden soil, may look and taste like kale, just as a child given a diet of sweets, chips and the occasional vitamin tablet, will still grow and look like a child. But looks aren't everything – it's what on the inside that counts. Fortunately, nature provides everything needed for nutrient-rich plants, meaning you don't need to rely on anything created in a lab.

The importance of healthy soil

Soil is a unique, living, breathing, moving, underground environment, as complex and as diverse as the one we inhabit above ground. It's teeming with micro-organisms including bacteria, fungi, protozoa and microscopic worms, and scores of larger creatures like millipedes and earthworms.

Like a finely tuned orchestra, these organisms work together to produce a complex masterpiece. But take out the string section, or zap some of these microbes with alien chemicals and things start to go wrong. Try to beat nature at its own game with synthetic compounds and the harmony is lost, the rhythm is disturbed.

Soil is a perfectly composed symphony of elements, with everything needed for plants to thrive. All you need to do is support it, like a sympathetic conductor, who steers but doesn't override the original composition.

Yet as plants grow they take nutrients from the earth which need to be replaced. Fortunately, we can use nature to do this job for us, without needing to resort to anything out of a plastic container.

What do fruit and vegetables need to grow?

In school, you probably learnt that plants need water, warmth, air, light and nutrients to grow. Which is of course, correct. But for super growth leading to nutrient-packed plants, crops also need a healthy balance of the right minerals, the most important of which are nitrogen, phosphorus and potassium, or N, P and K, to give them their chemical symbols. All plants need all these minerals, and others, but in different amounts.

NITROGEN ☼

Nitrogen promotes leaf growth and helps plants to grow greener and faster. Nitrogen can be depleted over time by plants, or by being washed away, and is the mineral needed in greatest quantities. Plants lacking in nitrogen will look sickly and yellow, with limited growth. However, that doesn't mean you need to marinade your crops in nitrogen – too much of a good thing isn't good either, and an excess can lead to too much foliage at the expense of something edible, as well as other problems. As nitrogen stimulates growth, plants need it most during spring and summer and some crops such as cauliflower, Brussels sprouts and other brassicas, are particularly nitrogen-hungry. Good sources include urine, animal manure and nettle tea (see the next section.)

PHOSPHOROUS ☼

Phosphorous is good for root growth and disease resistance and helps plants to grow strong. Most soils, especially those that contain plenty of organic matter, have adequate amounts of phosphorous, so it shouldn't be necessary to add any extra and deficiencies are uncommon. However, if the pH of soil is too high or too low, phosphorous may be locked up. Lack of phosphorous can result in weak plants with a feeble root system, and purple-tinged leaves. Too much phosphorous can block the absorption of other minerals.

POTASSIUM ☼

Potassium, which is sometimes called potash, is needed for plants to flower and produce fruit. It also helps protect plants against disease. Potassium is especially useful for fruiting plants, like tomatoes, as it boosts sugar levels in the plant, promoting bumper crops of the best tasting, sweetest fruit. So a lack of potassium may result in low levels of fruit, with a less than spectacular flavour. Don't overdo it, though; too much potassium can stop other minerals like magnesium from being absorbed, and this too can lead to poor growth and other issues. Good organic sources of potassium include seaweed and comfrey (see the next section.)

A BIT OF EVERYTHING ☼

To remain healthy, plants need a good supply of nitrogen, phosphorous and potassium, as well as other minerals including calcium, sulphur and magnesium, and a number of micronutrients, or trace elements which are needed in smaller quantities. All these minerals are found in good, healthy soil. So, in order to grow the tastiest, most nutrient-dense fruit and veg, it helps to understand your soil and how to replenish it. Treat it nicely and it will repay you generously.

Get to know your own soil

To bring out the best in your plants, it's good to know what you are planting them in. There are several different soil personalities – or types – from light-hearted and easy to get along with, to heavy going and intense. All have their pros and cons, you just need to play to their strengths and address any issues.

Sandy

Sandy soils have larger particles than other types of soil. This makes it easy to dig and quick to warm up in spring. Sandy soil doesn't tend to get waterlogged, as the loose texture means rain drains quickly through it. The downside is that nutrients are easily washed away and sandy soil tends to get dry in summer. Covering this type of soil with organic material helps it to retain both nutrients and moisture. Root crops like carrots and parsnips do particularly well in sandy soils.

Clay

Clay soils are made up of tiny particles with a tendency to clump together. If in doubt, ask your back – clay soils are heavy and hard to dig! On a positive note, this type of soil gets an A grade for retaining moisture and nutrients, so hungry crops like broccoli and cauliflower will thrive.

A soil that is rich in clay can easily become waterlogged, so avoid trampling on it and compressing it after rain. But at least there will be less watering to do during summer. Clay soils are slow to warm up in spring so don't be tempted to sow your seeds too early, as they won't germinate. The upside of this is that the heat is retained for longer into autumn. Towards the end of the year, when the harvest is over and the ground is still soft, dig in some organic matter to improve the structure of clay soil and make it more workable. Your vertebrae will thank you.

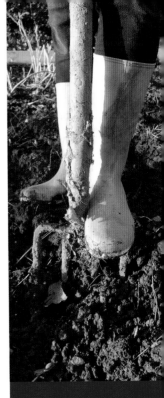

WHAT IS SOIL?

Soil is made up of minerals (rock, sand, clay and silt) plus air, water and organic matter from dead plants and animals. This organic matter is decomposed into humus thanks to the presence of all those worms and microbes. It is during this essential process that the vital nutrients that plants need for healthy growth are released into the soil. Not all soils are created equal, though, so it helps to work out what kind of soil you have before getting stuck in.

Silty

Silty soils are made of small, silty grains. Like sandy soils, this type of soil is easy to dig and free-draining, but can be low in nutrients. It is also easily compacted after heavy rain, so it helps to cover the surface with a blanket of organic material like compost.

Loamy

If you have this type of soil, count yourself lucky. Loam soil is a perfect balance of clay, sand and silt. It is easy to work with and holds water and nutrients well without becoming clogged up or waterlogged.

Multiple personality

In reality, most soil doesn't fit neatly into one category and is likely to be a combination of all or some of the above, with one type of particle dominating.

The quickest way to work out your soil's personality is to get your hands dirty. Roll some into a ball and if the soil sticks together easily and holds its shape, then it's high in clay. If it feels gritty and falls apart easily, it's sandy. In the end, it doesn't really matter what type of soil you have. As long as you look after it, stuff will grow. And don't worry too much about the weeds; they will grow too but their growth most likely indicates the presence of nutrients.

So how do you turn your sand, clay, silt or loam into super soil? Fortunately, there are all sorts of ways to cultivate the perfect medium in which to grow super foods. From making your own compost, to brewing your own nettle tea and even taking advantage of your own bodily fluids, it all comes down to working with nature.

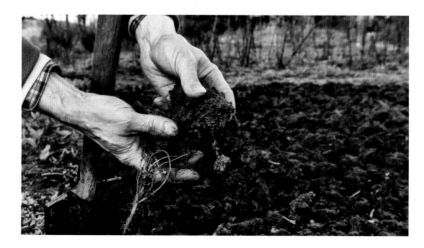

The quickest way to work out your soil's personality is to get your hands dirty ...

COMPOSTING – Garden compost

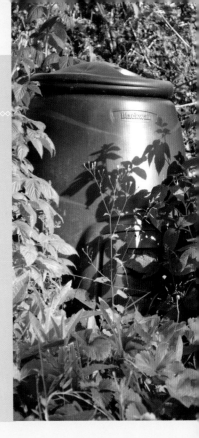

Home composting forms the groundwork to organic gardening and is essentially just a form of recycling. Most people recycle glass and plastic, so why not kitchen and garden waste too? As plants grow they take nutrients from the earth. When we eat these plants, the nutrients are absorbed by our own bodies.

But anything left over – the leaves, the stems, the bits the kids chuck on the floor – can be rotted down to provide compost, allowing all the remaining nutrients to be returned to where they came from. It saves time and money and will do your soil the world of good.

Making compost is a bit like making soup – you chuck in the right ingredients, mix them together and let them simmer – or in this case, let the micro-organisms get on with the decomposition process.

Choose your bin

To start with you will need a decent sized receptacle in which to dump all your waste. There are plenty of options to suit every garden and budget, from the familiar Tardis-style plastic compost bins, to hot bins and even solar-powered contraptions. Alternatively, you can make your own compost bin out of wooden pallets, or fence posts and chicken wire.

Stand your compost bin on bare soil. This allows moisture to get out and worms and other organisms to get in. If you don't have a spare patch of earth, then add a layer of soil to the bottom of the bin. You could introduce some worms too.

Choose a site with a bit of shade that's not at the mercy of the elements, as the process works best with consistent temperatures. It can take anything from six months to two years to make compost, though things speed up during the summer.

The compost is ready when it's dark and crumbly and smells slightly sweet. By this stage it will be full of plant nutrients. Dig it into the ground during the autumn to help improve the fertility and condition of the soil. Or use it as a mulch in spring and summer, spreading it around the base of plants to help conserve moisture and suppress weeds, while nourishing the crops.

Useful tips

☼ Use a garden fork to turn the compost over every month or so. This can be a bit tricky but it helps to aerate the heap which speeds up decomposition.

☼ Keep the compost damp, but not too wet. It shouldn't be slimy.

☼ If possible, try to have at least two compost bins, one full of ready to use rotted down matter, and another that you keep topping up with waste. The decomposition process works best when the bin is full, so try to fill it up as quickly as possible.

☼ You can speed up the composting process by providing an extra dose of nitrogen. Good sources include nettle and comfrey leaves and used pet bedding, for example from chickens, rabbits, guinea-pigs or hamsters.

☼ If you don't have any small animals to hand (or even if you do) the most convenient compost activator actually resides in your own bladder. Human urine is rich in nitrogen and perfect for speeding things up in the bin or on the heap - and think how much water you'll save by not having to flush. Although from a practical perspective, it can be easier to add this liquid gold via a bucket. Especially if you're a woman.

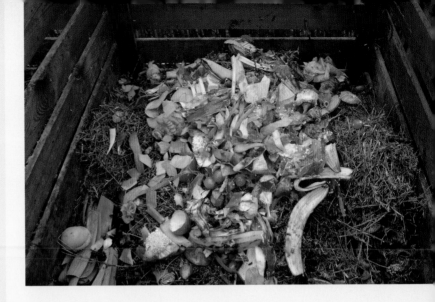

What to throw in a compost bin

Compost should be a roughly equal mix of wet greens (nitrogen-rich stuff) and dry browns (carbon-rich stuff.)

Greens:
- Fruit and vegetable peelings and waste
- Grass cuttings (but not too much) • Tea bags • Annual weeds

Browns:
- Scrunched up newspaper • Cardboard (not coloured)
- Empty loo rolls and egg boxes
- Woody prunings and twigs (chop or shred these before adding them)
- Straw

Other things to add:
- Crushed egg shells
- Natural fibres (cotton or wool)
- Ash from wood fires (not too much)

What not to add:
- Diseased plants
- Dairy, meat or fish products – this can lead to harmful bacteria and encourage rats
- Dog, cat or human faeces
- Perennial weeds – these will remain in the compost and return to the soil once you start using the compost
- Citrus (slow to break down and can be too acidic for worms)

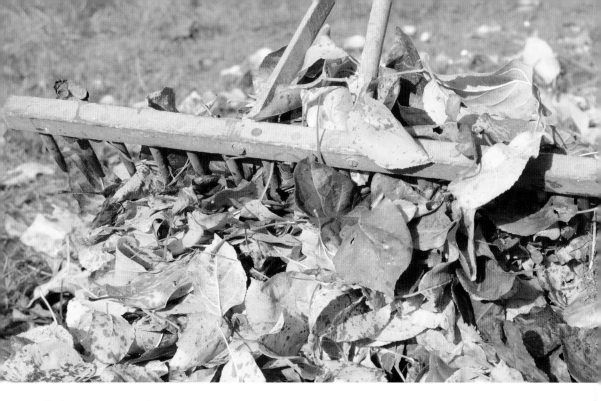

Other types of compost

Leaf mould

Despite the name, leaf mould isn't mould, but a compost made from decayed leaves, also known as 'gardener's gold'. It isn't as rich in nutrients as other types of compost but is excellent for improving the structure of soil and for spreading on the surface as a mulch. It can also be used as potting compost.

To make leaf mould, simply scoop up piles of fallen leaves in autumn and dump them into a wire enclosure. The easiest way to make one of these is to hammer four posts into the ground, then wrap some chicken wire or mesh around the outside of the frame and fix it to the posts, so it looks like a square cage. The mesh will stop the leaves from blowing away, while allowing the air to circulate. Top up the pile whenever there are more leaves to collect but avoid using those from busy roads which may contain pollutants.

Alternatively, you can you can make leaf mould in thick black bin bags. Simply punch some holes in the bags for ventilation, fill them with leaves, sprinkle on some water, and tie the bags at the top. Then leave in a cool, dark place – a shed is ideal – for a couple of years.

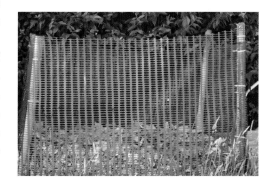

It takes about two years for the leaves to rot down completely. By this stage it will be dark and crumbly and can be used to condition the soil, or as potting compost. If you can't wait that long, leaf mould can also be used as a mulch after just one year, to help keep down weeds, and slowly improve the soil.

Bokashi

Another way to turn kitchen waste into compost is to ferment it. Strange as it sounds, the technique, which was developed in Japan in the 1980s, has recently started to catch on elsewhere.

It involves placing food waste (fish, meat, bones, the lot) in a special airtight bucket and adding extra-efficient micro-organisms, known as EM.

The waste ferments within a matter of weeks and you can then dig it into the soil, or add it to a compost bin. The system is fast, odourless and compact and you can recycle food that you can't add to a normal compost bin. The downside is you need to buy the bokashi kit in the first place.

Farmyard manure

Well-rotted horse manure is full of nutrients and is a valuable asset for any veg patch or allotment. If you don't have your own thoroughbred, riding stables, farms and police stables, often sell or give away manure. If you're really lucky, some allotments even have the stuff delivered.

Worms and their poo

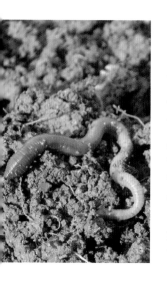

Worms are an essential part of the garden. As well as aerating the soil, they break down organic matter and leave behind worm casts, or waste, which are full of nutrients that enrich the soil and promote healthy plant growth. Charles Darwin concluded that life on earth would be impossible without worms. Healthy soil should be positively squirming with worms, and you can encourage them by adding plenty of organic matter for them to chomp on. And avoid using a rotavator, as, contrary to popular belief, a severed worm doesn't metamorphose into twins! Even digging carries a threat, so it's better to use a fork rather than a spade to minimise casualties.

You could go even further and invest in a wormery, or make your own worm hotel. A wormery is a great way of turning kitchen waste into high quality compost and is particularly good if you don't have much space, as they take up much less room than a normal compost bin, and benefit from having small amounts of waste added at a time.

Green manure

Green manures are plants grown specifically to benefit the soil and prevent erosion. Many absorb nitrogen from the air, which is released into the soil when the plant is dug into the ground. Green manures are also known as 'cover crops' as they are used to cover bare soil and suppress weeds. As such, they are often sown in autumn and grown over winter, before being dug into the soil in spring. Good ones to grow include crimson clover and grazing rye.

Liquid fertilisers

Compost and manure provide the backbone of organic gardening and will do wonders for your soil. But some greedy crops like broccoli, tomatoes, cauliflowers and strawberries will benefit from an extra nutritional boost in the form of a healthy drink, or liquid feed. But why buy commercial fertilisers, when you can save money and resources by rustling up home-brewed liquid feeds in your own back garden, as easily as whipping up a smoothie?

Nettle tea

Never mind the nasty rash, this is one weed you can turn to your advantage. Not only are nettle leaves edible – and delicious in soup and pasta – they also make a fantastic tonic for plants, due to their high mineral content. Nettles are especially rich in nitrogen which is particularly important for leafy crops, salads and young plants.

To make nettle tea, fill a bucket or large container (ideally one that has a lid) with fresh nettles, squashing them down so you can pack lots in. Wear a pair of thick gloves for this (nettles are horribly good at stinging through thin ones.) Fill the bucket with water so that all the nettles are submerged, cover with a lid, or plastic bag, and leave to stand for three weeks - after which time the concoction will absolutely stink!

Dilute with about ten parts water, to one part nettle tea, and use every couple of weeks as an instant tonic for plants.

Comfrey tea

If there's one thing plants love more than nettle tea, it's comfrey tea – and if you thought nettle tea reeked, this is even worse!

Comfrey, which has thick leaves and blue flowers, isn't as commonplace as nettles, but it's worth growing for its fertiliser properties alone. This gardening hero contains the holy grail of minerals needed for healthy plant growth: potassium, phosphorus (or potash) and nitrogen. It's a particularly good source of potassium which is essential for fruiting plants like tomatoes, strawberries, peppers and cucumbers. Treat these plants to a glug of comfrey tea once a week once fruit is starting to form and you will soon notice the difference.

You can make comfrey tea in the same way as nettle tea – or even use both together for a blended brew with extra nitrogen – then use the diluted liquid to give your plants an instant pick me up.

You can grow your own comfrey from seed or root cuttings. There are lots of different varieties but the best one to use as a fertiliser is Bocking 14, which doesn't set seed, so won't take over.

You can also use comfrey leaves as a mulch, or add them to the compost bin as a compost activator.

Seaweed

Seaweed has recently enjoyed something of an image shift – from slimy weed to superfood and culinary delicacy. But gardeners have known about its magical properties for centuries. Seaweed is packed with nutrients, including nitrogen, potassium, phosphate and magnesium, as well as those trace elements that are often lacking in commercial fertilisers, but needed by plants in small quantities.

Liquid seaweed is widely sold in garden centres but if you can manage to get hold of the fresh stuff you can make your own for nothing. If you don't live close to the sea, consider taking a spare bucket or two the next time you go on holiday. Check it's okay with the council or land owner before taking seaweed from the beach, and don't remove it from any conservation areas.

To make a liquid feed from seaweed, simply leave it to stew inside a bucket of water for a week or more, then use it to water plants, or spray onto the leaves every couple of weeks. The longer you leave it, the stronger it will get, so dilute it until it's the colour of weak tea.

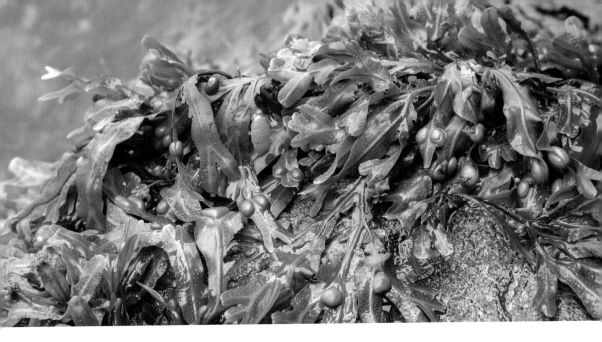

You can also dig fresh seaweed into the soil like manure, use it as a mulch, or add it to the compost bin. Whatever you do with it, you will be rewarded with super plants.

Wee

As well as adding urine to the compost bin, it can also be used as a liquid feed for your hungriest crops. Not only is it completely free, it's also available on tap. Urine is rich in nitrogen so it's good for boosting plant growth, and leafy crops. Dilute it with about nine parts water and use it as a tonic every couple of weeks. Don't overdo it – too much of a good thing isn't good for plants either! And always water the soil, rather than the plant itself.

Crop rotation

Crop rotation is a bit like changing your bedding. If you never do it, it will end up thin, smelly and possibly harbouring a few unwelcome pests. And nobody wants bed bugs.

Soil is the same: if you grow the same crops in the same place every year, they will soon wear out the earth, stripping away much of the goodness and leaving it vulnerable to pests and disease.

The idea of crop rotation is to avoid growing plants from the same family in the same spot in consecutive years, and instead to move them around the plot like a very drawn out game of musical vegetables. You could just mix and match, but apart from being a bit muddly, it helps to group crops from the same family together because they will all have similar requirements. For example, leafy

The idea of crop rotation is to avoid growing plants from the same family in the same spot in consecutive years ...

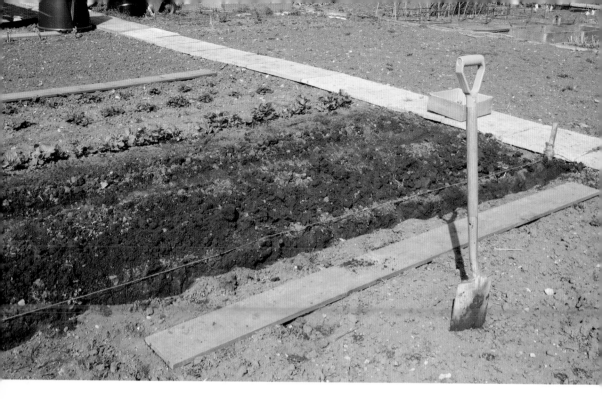

crops need lots of nitrogen, whereas beans and legumes, which make their own, need less.

Most crop rotation plans last three or four years, but it depends how much space you have and how many different kinds of plants you want to grow. For lots of gardeners, a four year plan is ideal.

How to work out a crop rotation plan

First, list all the crops you want to grow, then group them together into the following categories. Some fruits and vegetables aren't included, but don't worry about those for now.

- Alliums (onions, shallots, garlic, leeks.)
- Legumes (peas, beans and broad beans.)
- Brassicas (cabbages, cauliflower, Brussels sprouts, broccoli, kale etc.)
- Roots (potatoes, carrots, parsnips, beetroot.)

Next, divide your vegetable garden or allotment into four different sections. You don't have to create physical boundaries, just come up with a basic floor plan. Then jot it down on a piece of paper, so you don't forget it.

Now, decide which group of vegetables you want to grow in each section. You can grow them in any order you like, but it makes sense for plants which add nitrogen to the soil (beans and other legumes) to be followed by those that need it most, like broccoli and other members of the brassica family. Then once the brassicas have used up a hefty supply of nutrients it's a good idea to plant a less demanding crop like carrots in that area the following year, to give the soil a chance to recover. With this in mind, your plan might look like this:

Year One
Area 1: Root vegetables
Area 2: Brassicas
Area 3: Legumes
Area 4: Alliums

The following year you would just move everything on one place, so it would look like this:

Year Two
Area 1: Alliums
Area 2: Root vegetables
Area 3: Brassicas
Area 4: Legumes

In year three, you move everything along one place again, and the same in year four. So, by the fifth year, you are back to where you started. Simple!

Misfits
Some crops don't fit into the main families, so you can squeeze these in wherever there is space. These include things like lettuce, cucumbers, courgettes, squash and tomatoes, although it's best not to plant tomatoes with potatoes as they are from the same family and can spread blight, a dreaded fungal disease that can ruin two crops for the price of one.

Perennials
These are the plants that come back year after year – a bit like buy once, receive a free gift for the rest of your life. And as these plants remain in the same spot each year, they don't need including in a rotation system.

Examples include: asparagus, currant bushes, raspberries, rhubarb and strawberries, although strawberries will need to be replaced after about four years when they become less productive – a kind of short term perennial, if you like.

Bend the rules

☀ It doesn't matter if you don't stick to a completely rigid rotation plan. It's better to grow something, than leave an empty space.

The important thing is to remember what you've grown in each bed and try to grow something different there for the next two or three years. Your soil will thank you and hopefully your plants will reward you too.

Companion planting

Companion planting is a friendly way of trying to keep pests away from your precious fruit and vegetables, without having to use chemicals and pesticides. It involves growing certain plants together to help deter bad bugs, or to encourage 'good bugs' which eat the unwanted ones, a bit like employing a horticultural bodyguard. You can also grow mutually beneficial plants which help each other out for a win-win situation.

Companion plants can also offer physical help in the form of shade, support and nutrients, as well as providing a magnet for pollinating insects. And of course, growing flowers alongside your edibles adds that extra wow factor, too.

Here are some commonly used companion plants that will boost your garden's productivity and appearance, while keeping everything beautifully organic.

Nasturtiums

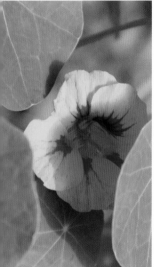

Nasturtiums are one of the easiest flowers to grow, so easy in fact that you may end up pulling some out because you've got too many. They are also one of the most useful companion plants as their pungent scent repels many insects, including whitefly, a common problem for tomato plants.

Nasturtiums also attract blackfly, which can attack bean plants. So plant nasturtiums as a sacrificial offering among your legumes and hopefully the bugs will choose the flowers and leave the beans alone.

To add to their talents, nasturtiums are also rich in mustard oils. This makes them highly attractive to the cabbage white butterfly, whose caterpillars can polish off an entire bed of brassicas overnight. So, plant some nasturtiums among your kale and broccoli and let them devour the flowers instead.

Poached egg plant

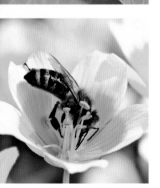

One of the best methods of organic pest control is to get predatory insects to the job for you. The aptly named poached egg plant, whose pretty yellow and white flowers resemble poached or fried eggs, attracts hoverflies, who love nothing more than assassinating aphids.

Leeks, onions, garlic and chives

Plant these strong-smelling members of the onion family near your carrots, or mix spring onion and carrot seed together. The onion smell masks the scent of the carrots, so the carrot fly doesn't know where to find them. In exchange, carrots planted with leeks can help deter the leek moth.

Herbs

Fragrant herbs like basil, mint, coriander and savory can help deter aphids, so dot them around your plot for a multi-layered approach. Even if it doesn't work, you'll still have a useful supply of kitchen ingredients. Mint is said to be particularly good for getting rid of ants, just tear up some leaves and scatter them wherever you have an infestation. However, mint can be quite invasive, so it's best to grow it in pots.

Fennel, dill and yarrow

Plants with clusters of tiny flowers like fennel, dill and yarrow are magnets for beneficial insects including tiny predatory wasps, lacewings, hoverflies and ladybirds. Attracting plenty of these into the garden will not only help with pollination but will also make a useful hole in the local aphid population.

Supportive plants

Companion planting can also be a means of providing physical support. For example, climbing beans can be grown up the sturdy stems of sweetcorn plants or sunflowers. And sprawling plants like squash and pumpkins can be grown underneath, so you get two or more harvests from one patch of soil, as one grows horizontally, and the others vertically. What's more, the large leaves of the squash plant help to suppress weeds and conserve moisture in the soil.

Wildflowers

Growing flowers alongside your super foods adds beauty and diversity to your plot. More importantly, it provides a magnet for flying insects who in their everyday pursuit of nectar will accidentally pollinate your crops just when you need it the most. Many crops rely on insect pollination in order to produce fruit, so the more bees and butterflies you can entice into your domain, the better. Just sprinkle a packet of wildflower mix over some soil and wait for the buzz – followed, hopefully, by bumper harvests.

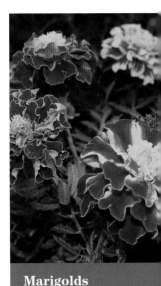

Marigolds (Tagetes patula) Like nasturtiums, French marigolds are very easy to grow and can be planted with most vegetables as their scent deters many insects. Again, they are often grown with tomatoes to repel whitefly. What's more, chemicals in the roots of marigolds can help suppress nematodes (microscopic worms that invade plant roots.)

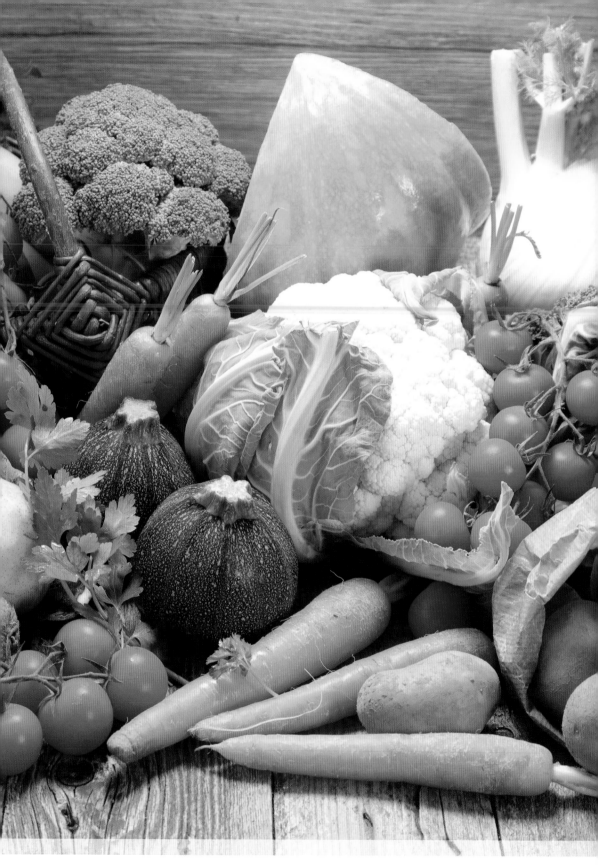

Part Two

This section contains all you need to know to grow a whole range of nutrient-packed fruit and vegetables in your own back garden, or allotment. Some crops can even be grown without a garden, as long as you have a few containers. You will also find information on the nutritional prowess of each crop, including the potential benefits of some of the most powerful and exciting plant compounds, or phytonutrients, found in even the most ordinary of foods. There is compelling evidence that eating a broad range of these chemicals can significantly lower the risk of cancer, heart disease and other conditions.

Of course, the whole point of growing delicious, healthy food is to enjoy eating it afterwards. So as well as information on how to grow an A-Z of super foods, you will find recipes to accompany each crop, bringing the joy of gardening into the kitchen. This isn't a diet book, so while many of the recipes are fantastically healthy, others are unapologetically indulgent. But after all that digging you deserve a treat!

If you have never grown anything before, gardening can seem like a whole new world, with its own mysterious rules and indecipherable language, inhabited by a green-fingered, green-wellied population. Fortunately, nothing could be further from the truth; you don't need to speak botany (or have a degree in it) to grow your own food. As long as you can read the instructions on a packet of seeds, you can make stuff grow. And as for green-fingers – just get a pair of gardening gloves.

In order to make this book accessible to both complete beginners and the already-initiated, I have tried to avoid using technical terms and jargon as much as possible. But just as it helps to have a few basic tools in your gardening arsenal – a fork, a trowel and a watering can – it can be useful to know a bit of the lingo, too. So here are a few terms that crop up from time to time:

Annual – a plant that germinates, flowers and dies (or is picked) within one ye ar. It is then sown again from seed the following year.

As long as you can read the instructions on a packet of seeds, you can make stuff grow ...

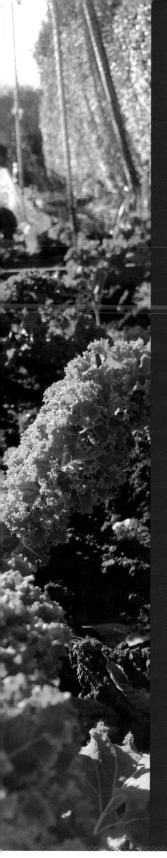

Bare-root – a plant that is removed from the soil while dormant and sold without being potted into a container. Fruit canes are often sold this way and are cheaper than container-grown plants.

Brassica – plants belonging to the cabbage family such as broccoli, kale and cauliflower.

Bolting – when a plant produces seeds or flowers too early, often making it inedible.

Cloche – a small glass or plastic cover that is placed over young plants to keep them warm. Shop-bought cloches are usually dome-shaped, or you can make you own from plastic bottles cut in half.

Hardening off – the process of moving indoor grown seedlings outside for a few hours each day and taking them in again at night. This gets them used to lower temperatures so they can then be planted permanently outside after about a week.

Intercropping – planting fast maturing crops in between slower growing ones.

Mulch/Mulching – spreading a layer of compost, manure or other organic matter over the soil, or around plants. This improves the soil and also helps to conserve moisture and suppress weeds.

Perennial – a plant that lives for more than two years. Many perennials such as raspberries, currants and artichokes will keep on growing year after year.

Pinch out – removing the growing tip of a plant by squeezing it between your finger and thumb, or snipping it off. This encourages the plant to grow in the direction you want.

Successional sowing – sowing small amounts of seed at regular intervals to ensure a continual harvest and avoid a large glut.

Thinning out – removing some seedlings or plants to give others more space to grow and reduce competition for light and nutrients.

Transplanting – moving a seedling or plant from one growing place to another, such as from a container into the vegetable patch.

Artichokes

♥ Love them

Not to be confused with the unrelated Jerusalem artichoke, the beautiful globe artichoke has been revered for its medicinal and digestive properties since the Greek and Roman times. Fast forward a couple of millennia, and it has re-emerged as a gourmet food, nutritional supplement and hangover cure combined – although don't count on this last one. It would take a mighty 'superfood' to undo the effects of too much wine, and unsurprisingly scientists have largely dismissed such claims.[5]

While they may not provide an antidote to alcohol, artichokes can help keep your liver healthy. The prickly-looking globes, which are actually edible flower buds, contain a high concentration of cynarin, a compound that increases the flow of bile. This helps to clear out harmful toxins as well as speed up the digestion of fats. What's more, they also contain another compound called silymarin, a flavanoid that can help protect the liver from toxins.

Artichokes are laden with other nutrients and antioxidants, too. In a comprehensive American study that rated more than 3,000 foods for their antioxidant content, artichoke was ranked fourth highest vegetable, and seventh overall.[6] Not bad for something that's basically a thistle.

Numerous studies have investigated the potential of artichokes to help prevent and control various diseases. There is evidence they may be useful for lowering cholesterol,[7,8] along with aiding digestive health and Irritable Bowel Syndrome, or IBS. Recent research has focused on the artichoke's anti-cancer properties, and results have shown that compounds found in the plant can lower the risk of

There is evidence they may be useful for lowering cholesterol, along with aiding digestive health and Irritable Bowel Syndrome ...

breast and other cancers, and kill abnormal cells.[9,10]

Of course, no food will ever provide a panacea against disease – if only there was such a thing as edible life insurance. However, there does seem to be a good case for including a few artichokes in your garden or allotment – and your diet.

On a cautionary note, artichokes, and especially supplements, are not recommended for people with existing liver, kidney or gallbladder problems.

❁ Grow them

Supermodels among the vegetable kingdom, artichokes are worth growing for their aesthetic value alone – although it would be a shame not to eat them, too. If space is limited in the veg patch, you can always plant them in a flowerbed or border, where they make stunning architectural plants.

The usual advice is to grow globe artichokes from small plants or 'offsets' as they are reputedly unreliable from seed. However, I've never experienced any problem with plants grown from seed. Luck? Maybe.

If you do take the seed route, sow them indoors in pots of compost in early spring. Harden the seedlings off a few weeks later

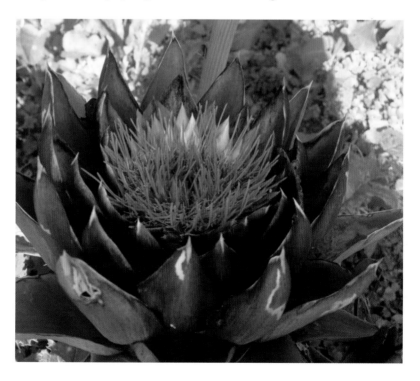

Artichoke in flower.

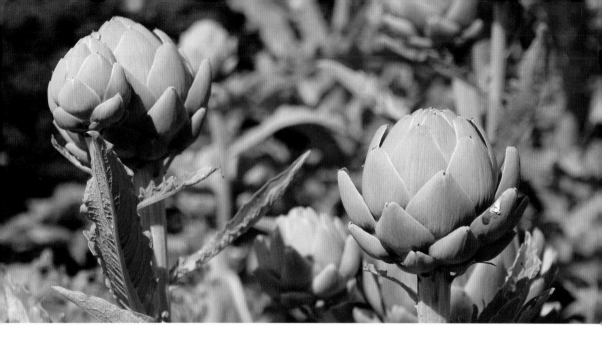

by placing them outdoors for a few hours each day for about week, before planting into the ground in May. Alternatively, you can buy young plants ready for planting straight outside, or take cuttings from established plants (see below.)

Artichokes need a sunny, sheltered spot with fertile soil and room to grow. Give them a good mulch of compost or manure after planting and leave about 90cm between plants.

Aftercare

In the first year, chop off any buds as soon as they appear. This is painful (for the gardener, not the plant) but you'll end up with a stronger plant in the long run. In autumn, cut off the old stems and leaves. In colder areas, cover the crown with straw.

Although globe artichokes are perennial plants and very low maintenance, they will need replacing after about four years. You can do this using the young plants that grow at the base of the main plant, called offsets. Carefully cut the new plant away by sliding a knife or sharp spade down the stem to separate it from the parent (leave some root attached) and then replant it.

Harvesting

Cut the highest globe first, while it's still fairly small and compact, followed by the lower ones. If you can restrain yourself, leave a couple of globes on the plant - they'll open up to produce the most incredible neon-blue feathery flowers. And the bees will appreciate your generosity.

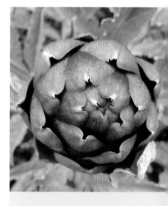

Varieties to try:

'Violetta di Chiogga' – attractive plants that crop well.

'Green Globe' – a reasonably hardy variety and a good choice for colder regions.

✌️💋 Eat them

IN GOURMET TERMS, the heart of the artichoke is considered the delicacy and this is often reflected in the price tag. But many of the nutrients are contained within the surrounding leaves, and these too are delicious.

Artichokes are rarely sold in their natural state, at least in the UK, and are more likely to be found swimming in a jar of oil or sitting on a pizza, so the most challenging thing about growing them can be knowing how to cook them afterwards. Fortunately, it's not difficult once you know how.

Preparation

Prepare the artichokes by pulling off the tough outer leaves and trimming the stalks to about 2cm. Then simply cook them whole, either by steaming or plunging into salted, boiling water. Cook until tender – around 10 to 20 minutes, depending on size. They are done when you can easily pull the leaves away from the stem.

There's no point trying to eat an artichoke politely. Just pull off a leaf, dunk it in something delicious like melted salty butter, or vinaigrette, and put it straight in your mouth – no cutlery required. Scrape off the soft green flesh with your teeth, discard the shell and repeat.

When you've worked your way through the leaves, remove the hairy bit in the middle – the aptly named choke – to reveal the final prize; the soft and delicate heart.

Stuffed artichokes (carciofi ripieni)

In Italy, where artichokes are an everyday vegetable, this is one of those classics that Nonna can whip up in minutes. For the rest of us it takes a bit more patience, but the end result is worth it. You could spruce up the filling with anchovies, olives and capers if you like, or stick to the original recipe.

- **1 globe artichoke per person**
- **Approx 2 tablespoons of breadcrumbs per artichoke** (depending on size of the globes)
  Don't be tempted to buy ready-made breadcrumbs, which taste nothing like real ones. Buy a loaf of unsliced bread, or a baguette in advance, let it dry out, then make your own breadcrumbs, using a fine grater or food processor.
- **A generous bunch of parsley, finely chopped**
- **A couple of cloves of garlic, finely chopped**
- **Salt and pepper**
- **A good splash of olive oil**
- **Half a lemon**

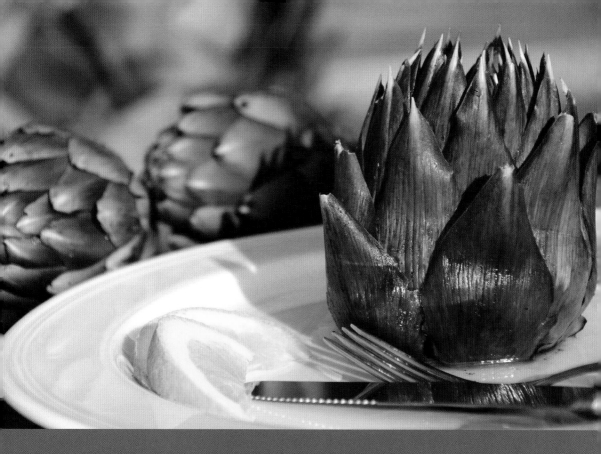

Method

• Prepare the artichokes by cutting off the stalks and removing the outer leaves, then rub them all over with lemon juice to prevent them from becoming discoloured. Gently tease the leaves apart with your fingers to create gaps between them and remove the hairy choke from each globe.

• Next, mix all the ingredients for the filling in a large bowl. The mixture should be fairly dry and not stick to the spoon.

• Stuff the artichokes with the mixture by pushing it into the gaps between the leaves with a teaspoon. Try to coat the inside of each leaf.

• Place the stuffed globes tightly together in a saucepan, then pour in enough water so that it comes half way up the sides of the artichokes. Simmer for around 20 minutes, or until tender. Eat as before by stripping away the leaves with your fingers and scraping off the flesh with your teeth.

Beetroot

♥ Love it

For all the hype surrounding beetroot, it is a true health giant among vegetables, packed with vitamins, minerals and antioxidants. Recent research indicates it may help prevent many diseases and chronic conditions, including high blood pressure, type 2 diabetes, dementia and cancer.[11] It could even improve your stamina in the gym.

The crimson globes are a good source of iron and folate (vitamin B9) manganese, magnesium, potassium and nitrates. The leaves are also tasty and highly nutritious, containing super amounts of vitamins A, C and K, as well as calcium and iron.

Many studies have shown that beetroot can help to lower blood pressure. This is because of the high concentration of nitrates, which the body naturally converts into nitrite, a chemical that can widen blood vessels and increase blood flow.[12] Hypertension (high blood pressure) affects more than a quarter of adults in the UK and can lead to heart disease and strokes if left untreated, so beetroot could play a valuable role as part of a healthy diet and lifestyle. What's more, beetroot contains a powerful compound called betacyanin – the stuff that gives it the distinctive colour. Betacyanin is a potent antioxidant and is believed to have cancer-fighting properties. And although more research is needed, it has been shown to slow the growth of breast and prostate tumours.[13]

Other studies have indicated that beetroot could help prevent dementia by improving blood flow to certain areas of the brain.[14] Similarly, it may boost exercise performance by allowing more oxygen to be delivered around the body.[15] No wonder a number of athletes have confessed to a healthy beetroot juice habit.

It might not turn you into an Olympian, but there is compelling evidence that beetroot does have many health benefits. It will even

it may boost exercise performance by allowing more oxygen to be delivered around the body ...

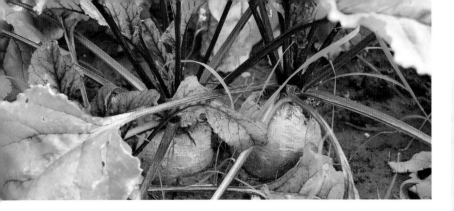

make your wee turn red – and there aren't many foods you can say that about. Just don't be alarmed when it happens!

✿ Grow it

Beetroot is exceptionally easy to grow and about as failproof as gardening gets. It does best in a sunny spot with light soil that has been given plenty of manure over the years, but it will generally survive anywhere. Just don't add manure directly before sowing as this will encourage the roots to fork.

The seed can be sown straight outside from March onwards once the ground has warmed up slightly and there is no further chance of frost. If the soil is waterlogged, then wait until conditions have improved.

Beetroot is usually sown in rows. You could stretch a length of string between two sticks to mark out a straight line, but an even easier way is to press something long and straight like a bamboo cane into the ground, to make a narrow channel about 2cm deep. This creates a ready-made groove into which to sprinkle your seeds.

Water the soil first, then sow the seed along the row, leaving about 5cm between each seed, then cover gently with soil. Or just scatter liberally and thin the seedlings out later on. Space additional rows about 25cm apart. For a continual harvest, sow new handfuls of seeds every few weeks until July.

Once the roots start to form, beetroot is fairly self-sufficient and only needs watering during very dry spells. All you really need to do is a bit of weeding now and then.

Harvesting

Once the roots reach golf ball size, from July onwards, pull them up by hand leaving others in the ground to grow bigger. Beetroot can be dug up and stored for several weeks in a cool, dark place, however unless you need the space, the roots will usually be fine left in the ground until you want to eat them.

Varieties to try:

'Bolthardy' – a reliable variety that is resistant to bolting. It can be sown early in the season, and will last until the following spring.

'Chioggia' – produces large beetroot which are striped on the inside, revealing striking red and white rings when sliced open.

'Rhonda' – delicious, sweet flavour, can be eaten as baby beet or grown to full size. Good bolting tolerance.

Growing tips

☀ If the ground is cold or it's been a hard winter, warm up the soil for a few weeks before sowing, by covering with plastic sheeting or garden fleece. Otherwise delay sowing until the weather improves.

⇌ Eat it

IN RECENT YEARS, beetroot has shaken off its vinegary, unpopular past to become a favourite among food lovers, chefs and the health-conscious. No longer confined to jars, this vibrant, versatile vegetable can be used in myriad ways. Young beetroot are delicious grated raw into salads or shaved into wafer-thin slices. The leaves can be added to salads, or cooked like spinach or chard.

To boil beetroot, leave a couple of centimetres of stalk at the top so the colour doesn't bleed and don't peel them. Simmer gently for around 50 minutes, depending on size. Once cooked, the skin will slide off with your fingertips (use the back of a knife, or wear rubber gloves if you don't want pink hands.) Beetroot are also perfect for roasting, either on their own or with other root vegetables.

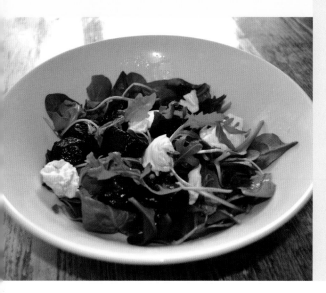

Roast beetroot, goats cheese and rocket salad

Sweet, tangy, peppery and colourful, what more could you ask of a salad? You could also add the beetroot leaves if they are still young and tender, or anything else you have growing like spinach or watercress.

Serves 4-6
- **600g raw beetroot**
- **4 tablespoons olive oil**
- **3 tablespoons balsamic vinegar**
- **200g goat's cheese**
- **A few handfuls of rocket, or other salad leaves**
- **Salt and pepper to season**

Method

- Preheat the oven to 200°C/180°C fan/gas 6.

- Scrub the beetroot, then cut into large wedges. Place a large piece of foil in a roasting tin and place the beetroot on top. Drizzle over the olive oil and balsamic vinegar, then season with salt and pepper. Scrunch the foil over to make a loose parcel that covers the beetroot.

- Roast for around 45 minutes, or until tender.

- Fold back the foil to uncover the beetroot, add the goat's cheese and return to the oven for 5 minutes or until the cheese becomes gooey.

- Remove from the oven, allow to cool slightly, then transfer to a bowl. Add the rocket, or other leaves, drizzle with a little more olive oil if you like, and serve.

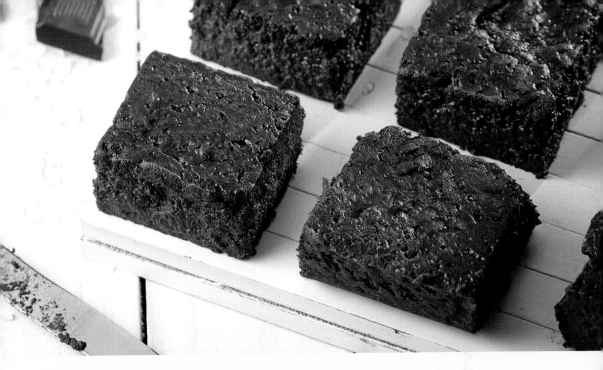

Secret beetroot brownies

Beetroot is naturally sweet and moist, making it an ideal ingredient for cakes and bakes. Add it either covertly or overtly to these brownies, depending on who you're feeding.

Makes approximately 20 squares
- **250g dark chocolate**
- **250g unsalted butter**
- **125g muscovado sugar**
- **125g caster sugar**
- **3 eggs**
- **150g plain flour**
- **25g cocoa powder**
- **225g beetroot, boiled and peeled, then mashed or pureed.**
- **A little icing sugar to finish** (optional)

Method
- Preheat the oven to 180°C/160°C fan/gas 4.

- Grease and line a baking tin, approx 20x25cm.

- Put the chocolate and butter in a large heatproof bowl and place it over a pan of simmering water, making sure the water doesn't touch the base of the bowl. Stir until melted.

- In a separate bowl, whisk the eggs and sugar until thick and creamy.

- Pour in the melted butter and chocolate and beat until smooth.

- Sift the flour and cocoa powder into the mixture and fold it in, followed by the beetroot. Stir the mixture gently.

- Pour into the tin and cook for around 25 minutes or until done. A skewer inserted into the middle should come out a bit sticky.

- Allow the brownies to cool in the tin. Dust with icing sugar, if you like, then cut into squares.

Beetroot preserve

This recipe was handed down by a French chef. As a relish, it goes fantastically well with cheese, cold meat, or oatcakes. But it's so good, you could just eat it on its own – straight out of the jar.

Makes several jars
- 1kg raw peeled beetroot, grated
- 300g fresh tomatoes, chopped
- 1 or 2 cloves of garlic, finely diced
- 1 onion, finely sliced
- 1 small red pepper, finely sliced
- 50g caster sugar
- 12g salt
- 140ml vegetable oil
- 140ml white wine vinegar
- Black pepper

Method

- Gently heat the oil, then add the tomato, onion and pepper and cook for around 10 minutes. Leave to stand.

- Place the grated beetroot in a large, separate pan and cook over a low heat. When it starts to bleed, add the sugar and salt and cook slowly for another 10 minutes.

- Add the cooked tomato, onion and pepper to the beetroot. Pour in the vinegar and cover the pan with a lid. Cook on a low heat for about 45 minutes, stirring occasionally.

- Add a few grinds of black pepper and the garlic and leave to simmer for 10 minutes.

- Transfer to sterilised jars and close the lids. Turn the jars upside down, cover with a tea towel and leave until cool, to seal. The preserve will keep for a few months.

Blackcurrants

♥ Love them

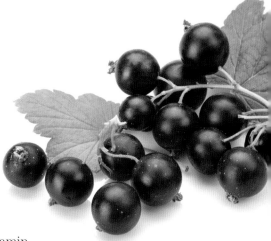

During the past decade, blackcurrants have been somewhat eclipsed by the trendier, arguably more palatable, blueberry, but along with that sharp burst of flavour, blackcurrants contain a bevy of vitamins, minerals and antioxidants that have been linked to many health benefits, from staving off colds and urine infections to guarding against cancer and chronic illnesses.

These inky little berries are amazingly rich in vitamin C – in fact, one serving of blackcurrants contains four times the amount of vitamin C found in the same weight of oranges.[16]

Blackcurrants are also one of the best sources of anthocyanins – the compounds that provide the deep purple pigment. As well as adding colour, anthocyanins are important antioxidants and are thought to help protect against ill-health, especially joint inflammation, heart disease and some cancers such as breast and ovarian.[17,18]

It has even been suggested that blackcurrants could help people with asthma. This is down to a natural chemical found in the berries called epigallocatechin. Although it's still early days, scientists have demonstrated that this compound can suppress lung inflammation in allergy-induced asthma, by working in harmony with the body's own natural defences.[19]

Blackcurrants may have other benefits too; one long-term study found that men who regularly consumed blackcurrants, and other flavanoid-rich foods and drinks including red wine, were significantly less likely to suffer from erectile dysfunction.[20]

If that's not enough to persuade you to sprinkle a few blackcurrants onto your breakfast cereal or fruit salad, then just think of all that immune-boosting vitamin C.

> These inky little berries are amazingly rich in vitamin C ...

❄ Grow them

Blackcurrants are perfectly suited to less than perfect climates, as they are hardy, unfussy plants. They will do best in fertile, slightly acidic soil, in full sun. But if this isn't available, they will put up

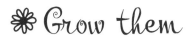

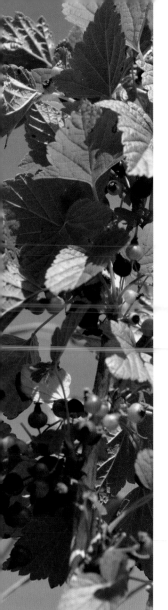

with most conditions, including a bit of shade, just as long as the soil isn't waterlogged.

The cheapest way to get started, is to buy bare-rooted plants. These can be planted between October and March, as long as the ground is not frozen. You can also buy pot-grown plants which can be planted at any time of the year.

How to plant

Dig a wide, deep hole and place the plant inside so that a good proportion of it is underground – around 6cm deeper than it was in the pot. This encourages strong growth and more fruit.

Water generously, then refill the hole with soil and press down firmly around the plant. It's a good idea to spread some mulch around the plant, such as compost or bark chips, to conserve moisture.

After planting, trim the shoots back to just above ground level to encourage new growth – if planting during summer time, wait until winter to do this. The bush will produce fruit the following year.

Pruning and aftercare

Prune blackcurrant bushes when they are dormant from late autumn to late winter, by cutting about one third of the older, thicker and darker stems down to ground and removing low branches and shoots.

In spring, place some compost or well-rotted manure around the base of the plant to enrich the soil and keep it damp.

Blackcurrants are very low maintenance and with simple pruning, mulching and watering, they should keep going for around 15 years.

Varieties to try:

'Ben Nevis' – frost and mildew-resistant with good flavoured fruit.

'Ben Sarek' – a heavy-cropping, dwarf bush, suitable for container growing.

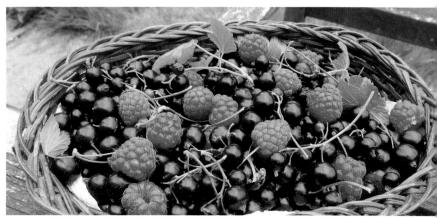

⋙ Eat them

RAW BLACKCURRANTS CAN be an acquired taste, but one that's well worth trying to acquire, given the health benefits. Otherwise, they work brilliantly in all sorts of jams, compotes, crumbles, cheesecakes and sponges. They can also be used to accompany strongly flavoured meats like duck and venison. If fruit and meat isn't your kind of fusion, this easy sorbet is a winner on a hot day.

Blackcurrant sorbet

You don't need an ice-cream maker to make this deliciously refreshing dessert. The addition of egg white gives it that smooth and light sorbet texture, although if you do happen to have an ice cream machine sitting around, feel free to omit the egg.

- **450g blackcurrants**
- **300ml water**
- **140g caster sugar**
- **1 egg white**
- **Fresh mint to garnish**

Method

• Place the blackcurrants and half the water in a saucepan and heat gently for about 10 minutes until soft. Puree in a blender, then sieve and allow to cool.

• Meanwhile, put the remaining water into a saucepan with the sugar and heat until the sugar has dissolved. Allow to cool completely.

• Mix the blackcurrants with the sugar syrup.

• Transfer to a freezer-proof container and place in the freezer until mushy. Whisk with a fork to soften it a bit more.

• Whisk the egg white until stiff, mix into the semi-frozen mixture to make it fluffy. Return to the freezer and leave until solid.

• Remove from the freezer 10 minutes before needed and serve with a sprig of mint.

Blackcurrant liqueur

I'm not suggesting this joyful brew is any way virtuous. Drink in *ahem* moderation. Unless you're under 18 of course – in which case leave out the vodka.

- 1kg blackcurrants
- 1 litre of vodka
- 500g sugar
- 150ml water

Method

• Wash the blackcurrants, then crush them to a pulp using the end of a rolling pin, or whizz them up in a blender.

• Transfer the purple mush to a large storage jar and add the alcohol.

• Seal and leave in a dark place for about four months. Give it all a good shake now and then.

• When those four months are finally up (write it on a calendar if you're likely to forget) strain the liqueur through a muslin into a clean bowl.

• Heat the sugar and water in a small saucepan until the sugar has dissolved. Allow to cool, then pour the syrup into the liqueur and stir.

• Transfer into clean bottles, seal, and put them into hibernation for another few weeks, somewhere dark and cool. The longer you wait, the better it tastes.

• You can drink the liqueur as it is, or mix with white wine to make a Kir, or add a splash to Prosecco or champagne to make Kir Royal. On the remote chance there's any left by December, a bottle of your home-made brew also makes a lovely Christmas present.

Blueberries

♥ Love them

Since bursting onto the superfood scene, blueberries have received rave reviews for their widely touted health benefits. It's claimed they can not only fight cancer and other diseases, but improve brain power and memory too. You could be forgiven for wondering how we ever survived without them!

Despite the hype, it's fair to say that blueberries are a super source of antioxidants. This is due to the rich concentration of anthocyanins, which provide the purple pigment. However, it's worth remembering that blueberries aren't the only anthocyanin stars; blackberries, blackcurrants, cherries, strawberries, aubergines, and many other red and purple coloured fruits and vegetables are all excellent sources, too.

Anthocyanins are part of the flavonoid family and have powerful antioxidant properties, helping to protect cells against free radicals – those notorious molecules that can damage our DNA, leading to ageing and disease. Many studies have been carried out to examine whether the anthocyanin content in blueberries can stave off this process. One large study found that women who ate three or more portions of blueberries and strawberries a week were 32 per cent less likely to have a heart attack than women who rarely ate them.[21] Other studies have indicated that blueberries may help lower blood pressure, although the evidence is still inconclusive.

Blueberries may also help keep our brains healthy. Researchers from Reading University in the UK found that primary school children displayed higher levels of memory and concentration skills after drinking high strength wild blueberry juice, compared to an alternative drink.[22] Although research is ongoing, it seems apparent that these little purple gems are not only delicious, but extremely nutritious too.

> Blueberries are a super source of antioxidants ...

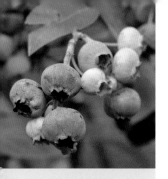

Growing tips

☀ Choose a sunny, sheltered spot.

☀ Keep the soil damp at all times and try to use rainwater as much as possible since tap water can make the soil less acidic.

☀ Once plants are three years old, prune every winter by removing old, dry wood.

☀ Cover the plants with netting once the berries emerge to stop the birds eating them all.

Varieties to try:

'Herbert' – produces lots of tasty, large berries with a sweet flavour.

'Bluecrop' – a popular variety and a heavy cropper.

'Nui' – produces huge berries for extra 'wow' factor.

❋ Grow them

Blueberries' exceptional health benefits are matched only by their exceptional price tag. And given that it's possible to polish off a punnet in less time that in takes to open the lid, it makes healthy financial sense to grow your own.

Although blueberry plants are easy to care for, they will only produce fruit in acid soil. This is also needed for rhododendrons, camellias and heather to flourish, so if you've got any of these growing in your garden you could be in luck. Otherwise, you can check the pH of your soil with a simple testing kit, sold in garden centres. For blueberry plants to thrive, the pH needs to be lower than 5. If it's higher, you can try to lower it by adding sulphur dust, or organic matter like pine needles, leaf mould, bark chippings or home-made compost. Realistically, this is a case of trial, time and error (mainly error, I have found) and it's often easier to grow blueberries in containers. Fortunately, they will do very well in large tubs filled with ericaceous (acid) compost, which is widely sold in garden centres.

Bare-root blueberry plants can be planted into the ground while they are still dormant between November and March. Container-grown plants can usually be planted all year round.

Although some blueberries will bear fruit on their own, it pays to grow a couple of different varieties to ensure good pollination and a heavier crop.

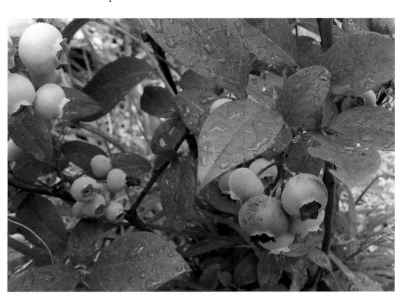

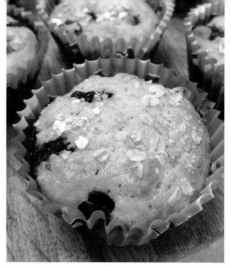

Eat them

THERE SEEMS TO be little point in cooking blueberries when they are so sweet and more-ish picked and eaten straight from the plant. If you have children, it's unlikely you will have any left anyway, but in the unusual event of a surplus, these muffins are a doddle to whip up.

Blueberry, oat and yoghurt muffins

Makes approximately 24 smallish muffins.

- **240g plain flour**
- **100g porridge oats, plus a little extra for sprinkling**
- **120g unsalted butter**
- **2 large eggs**
- **250g natural yoghurt**
- **225g golden caster sugar**
- **2 teaspoons baking powder**
- **300g blueberries**

Method

• Preheat the oven to 190°C/170°C fan/gas mark 5.

• Line muffin tins with paper cases.

• Melt the butter and allow to cool, then whisk in the eggs and yoghurt.

• Combine the dry ingredients and stir into the wet mixture, being careful not to over mix, then fold in the blueberries.

• Spoon the mixture into cases and sprinkle a few oats over the top of each muffin.

• Bake for around 25 minutes or until golden and cooked.

Blueberry Eton-ish mess

This recipe is so simple, you can't even call it cooking – unless you make your own amaretti biscuits, that is. I don't.

- Serves 6
- **300g fresh blueberries**
- **500g Greek-style yoghurt**
- **100g amaretti biscuits**
- **A splash of Amaretto liqueur** (optional)
- **Runny honey to finish**

Method

• Place 250g of the blueberries in a bowl with the Amaretto if using. Squash slightly with a fork. Tip in the yoghurt and stir.

• Roughly smash the amaretti biscuits, then fold these into the yoghurt mixture.

• Spoon into glasses or small bowls. Top with the remaining blueberries and drizzle some honey over each one.

Broad beans

♥ Love them

Broad beans are one of the oldest cultivated crops in the UK and have a been a Mediterranean staple for centuries, stretching back to the ancient Egyptians, Greeks and Romans. After dipping out of popularity for a while, these pearly legumes are on the up again.

Like other beans, they provide a double whammy of protein and fibre – one of the best combinations for avoiding hunger pangs and sugar cravings – along with hiding the biscuit tin. They are also a good source of vitamins C, A, B1, B2 and folate, and are rich in minerals, including magnesium, potassium, iron, copper, phosphorous and manganese.

To top it all, broad beans are a natural source of an amino acid called L-dopa, which the body converts into dopamine, a neurotransmitter that plays a role in mood regulation, sex drive and movement. It has been suggested that eating broad beans may help alleviate symptoms of depression, however, further research is needed. L-dopa is also used as a treatment for Parkinson's Disease, and there is hope that broad beans could potentially play a role in treatment, without the side effects of drugs.[23]

Alongside all the benefits, broad beans come with their own health warning. The beans, which are also known as fava beans, can cause a potentially dangerous reaction in people who suffer from favism, a rare inherited condition found predominantly among people of Mediterranean origins.

> Like other beans, they provide a double whammy of protein and fibre ...

❋ Grow them

Broad beans are childishly easy to grow. Another selling point is that you can plant them in the autumn and then pick them the following spring, before most crops have even got off the ground. This makes them a welcome filler during that awkward hungry gap. And of course, home-grown broad beans are miles better than shop-bought ones, without having travelled any actual miles.

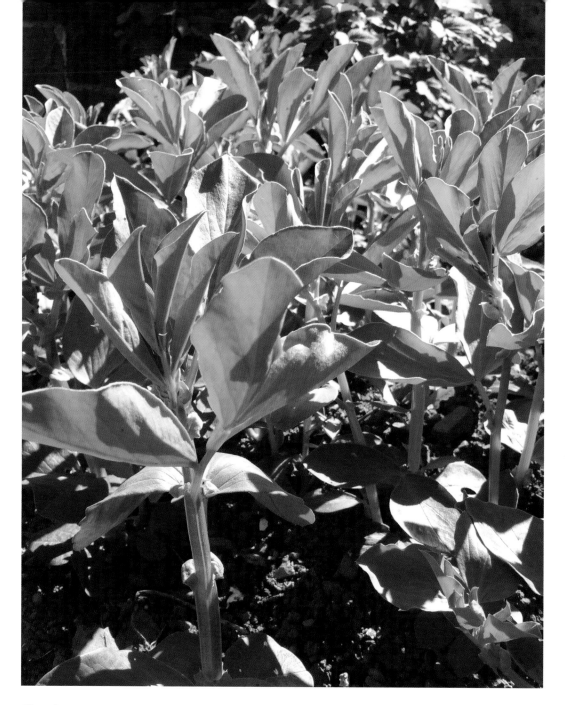

Sowing

For the earliest crops, broad beans can be sown in October or November. In colder areas, you might need to sow them under a cloche, or cover. It's also worth planting extra seeds as casualties are likely to be higher at this time of year. Alternatively, you can plant them in spring like most other crops.

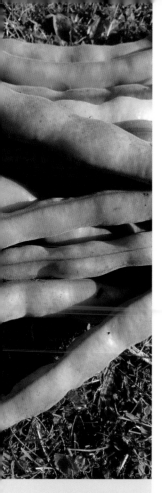

Whenever you choose to plant broad beans, it helps to enrich the soil by digging in some compost or manure, if possible. Rake the soil until it's fine and crumbly, then plant the seeds about 5cm deep and about 20cm apart, then cover them over with soil.

Broad beans can also be started off in pots, or empty toilet rolls, and transplanted into the ground once they have developed into seedlings. This is good if you like a bit more control over your seeds, but not so good if you want to save time.

Aftercare

Broad beans sometimes need propping up with sticks to keep them off the ground. This is especially true for taller varieties or those grown in exposed areas. Growing plants in blocks rather than rows also provides some support as the plants will help each other up to stand up. Once the first pods appear, pinch off the growing tip at the top of the plant to encourage the production of beans. These tips can also be eaten.

Keep the plants well watered and the soil free from weeds.

Harvesting

Broad beans are best eaten young, when they are sweet and tender and before the pods start to bulge. The lowest pods will be ready to pick first. Don't leave them on the plant too long or the beans will become tough and bitter.

After harvesting, cut the plants down to ground level but don't pull them up, as the roots help to 'fix' nitrogen into the soil. Dig them in at a later date, then capitalise on the added nitrogen by growing nutrient-hungry crops like brassicas in the same spot the following year.

Problems and troubleshooting

Birds – if pigeons and the like are a nuisance, you may need to cover your seeds with netting.

Blackfly – have an annoying fondness for broad beans and often cluster around the growing tips of the plants. The best solution is to pinch off these shoots along with the blackfly. This also concentrates the plant's energies into producing pods.

Chocolate spot – this is a fungal disease that leaves brown spots on the leaves. There's not much you can do, except try to leave enough space between plants for the air to circulate.

Varieties to try:

'Aquadulce Claudia' – a very hardy and popular variety. One of the best for autumn sowings.

'The Sutton' – a dwarf variety, good for early spring sowings, small spaces, pots and windy sites. Can also be grown under cover in autumn.

'Express' – a fast growing variety for sowing in spring.

👄 Eat them

THERE'S NO GETTING away from it, broad beans can be a bit of a faff to prepare, as they need releasing from not just one, but two layers of wrapping. As well as the communal outer pods, each individual bean is encased in its own skin. However, if the beans are young and fresh the skins are perfectly edible, so just leave them on. For beans that have passed the first flush of youth, double peeling might be necessary. Fortunately, children seem to quite enjoy this job, so if you have any to hand round them up to help with podding.

Preparation

Split open the pods and turf out the beans, then plunge them into a pan of boiling, salted water for a minute or so to soften the outer membranes. Rinse the beans under cold water, then pinch them between your fingertips until they pop free of their skins. A bit like squeezing a spot, only more appetising.

Your naked beans are now ready to cook and are brilliantly versatile. Steam, boil, or sauté them, stir into pasta or risotto, or try smashing them onto toast with garlic or spices. Broad beans can also be used instead of chickpeas to make hummus or falafels. Or simply dress them with olive oil, lemon juice and salt.

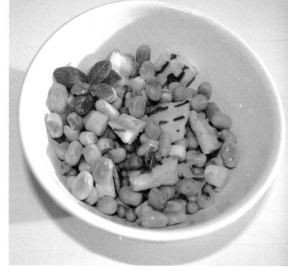

Broad bean, halloumi and mint salad

Serves 4
- **250g halloumi cheese**
- **400g broad beans, shelled weight**
- **200g peas**
- **Handful of spring onions, chopped**
- **Handful of mint leaves, torn**
- **A couple of glugs of olive oil**
- **Juice of half a lemon**
- **Salt and pepper to season**
- **Mixed salad leaves**

Method

• Steam the broad beans until just tender and cook the peas.

• Fry or griddle the halloumi then cut it into rough cubes.

• Combine the cheese, beans, peas, mint and spring onions.

• Whisk the olive oil, lemon juice and seasoning, or shake it all together in a jam-jar, then pour over the other ingredients and serve.

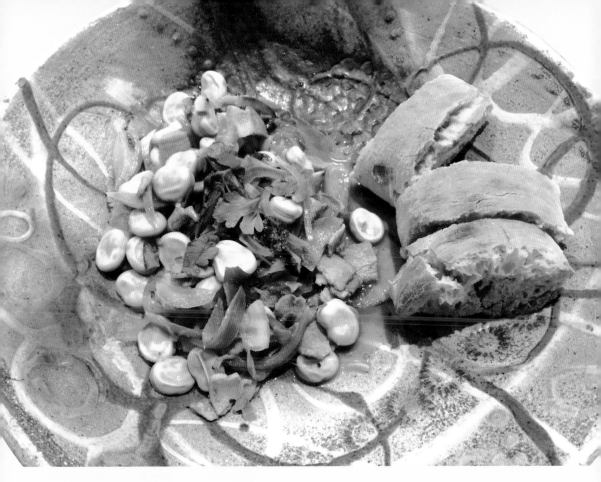

Warm broad beans with red onion and pancetta

Serves 4
- **550g broad beans, shelled weight**
- **130g pancetta cubes**
- **2 red onions, finely sliced**
- **2 tablespoons olive oil**
- **A handful of parsley, chopped**
- **200ml white wine**
- **water**
- **Salt and pepper to season**

Method

• Heat the oil in a large saucepan and fry the onion over a medium heat for a couple of minutes.

• Add the pancetta and cook until it starts to brown.

• Add the broad beans and stir.

• Pour in enough water so that everything is covered, then add the wine, parsley and seasoning.

• Cover and leave to simmer over a low heat for 10-15 minutes, or until done, stirring from time to time.

• Remove the lid, turn the heat up and cook for a few minutes to reduce the liquid, stirring well.

• Serve with crusty bread.

Broccoli

♥ Love it

Broccoli has been the subject of much hype in recent years and has been saddled with an eyebrow-raising list of super powers, with claims it can treat a catalogue of conditions including: cancer, heart disease, asthma, arthritis, diabetes and even autism. Of course, some of the headlines range from optimistic, to wildly overstated, but there is a compelling case that regularly eating broccoli as part of a healthy diet, could help reduce the risk of many chronic conditions and keep cholesterol in check.[24]

This household veg is packed with vitamins, minerals and antioxidants. Like many green vegetables, it contains more vitamin C than the equivalent amount of oranges – the popular benchmark by which all other vessels of vitamin C are measured. Broccoli is also a good source of iron, calcium, folate (vitamin B9) and vitamins K, B6, E and A (from beta-carotene.)

Of particular interest is a sulphur compound called sulforaphane. This natural plant chemical, which is also found in other brassicas like cauliflower and Brussels sprouts, has been widely studied and has been shown to have powerful anti-cancer and anti-inflammatory properties. Regular consumption of broccoli has been associated with a lower risk of many cancers, including those of the breast, lung, prostate, pancreas and colon. Sulforaphane has been shown to kill cancer stem cells and slow down tumour growth and is being studied for its ability to delay or block various forms of cancer with promising early results.[25]

It has even been suggested that broccoli may help improve the symptoms of autism. One small trial found that boys and young men who were given sulforaphane for 18 weeks, showed improved social interaction and verbal communication and decreased abnormal behaviour, compared to those who were given a placebo.[26]

Although further research is needed to harness broccoli's full potential, it seems verdantly clear that eating your greens will do you good, not just in the short term but hopefully in the long run, too.

It contains more vitamin C than the equivalent amount of oranges ...

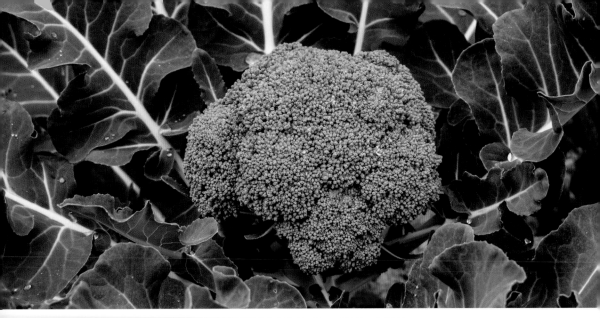

Calabrese, commonly known as broccoli.

❀ Grow it

There are two main types of broccoli; sprouting broccoli which consists of small purple or white florets on long stems and the familiar large green heads sold in supermarkets. This is actually calabrese, but for some confusing reason the heads are commercially labelled as 'broccoli'.

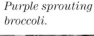

Purple sprouting broccoli.

Sprouting broccoli is much more expensive to buy than regular 'broccoli' or calabrese, and has slightly higher levels of vitamins and minerals, although both types are extremely good for you. So if you only grow one type of broccoli – and it does take up an awful lot of space – I'd recommend a sprouting one. Another bonus is that sprouting broccoli matures later, so is useful for filling that awkward hungry gap between winter and spring when other crops are sparse. (Although check the packet, as some varieties mature earlier.)

However, if you prefer the taste of calabrese and wouldn't splash out on posh gourmet types anyway, grow that!

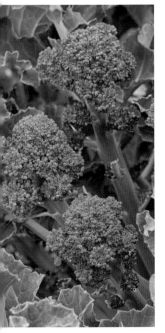

How to sow sprouting broccoli

Broccoli needs a nutrient-rich, firm soil, so it pays to dig in some well-rotted manure, or garden compost in the autumn before planting.

Start the seeds off in pots indoors in February or March, or directly outdoors in April. Transplant pot-grown seedlings into the ground when they are about 10cm tall, leaving 60cm between each plant. Don't be tempted to plant them any closer together – they'll hate you for it and will repay you with miserly pickings.

If the sight of empty soil makes you twitchy, sow a few cheeky salad leaves in between your broccoli seedlings. The salad will be ready to pick before the broccoli is fully grown, freeing up the space again. This is often called intercropping and is a great way to max out your plot. It's also far more productive than waiting for the weeds to make an appearance.

As the broccoli plants grow, build up the soil around the base of the stalks from time to time, to help them stand up in the wind.

Harvest from late winter once the spears are long enough to eat. Keep cutting them to encourage new heads to grow.

How to sow calabrese

Seeds can be sown straight into the ground from mid-March, although you can start them off in pots if you prefer, especially if slugs are on the prowl.

When sowing outside, start by creating a 1cm deep drill in the soil – an easy way to do this is to press a bamboo cane horizontally into the ground. Make sure the ground is damp before sowing, then sprinkle the seed along the row and cover over with a little soil.

Thin the seedlings out as they grow, to leave final gaps of 30cm between plants. Again, don't be tempted to let them rub shoulders – you'll just end up with claustrophobic, unproductive plants.

Calabrese can be harvested in summer and autumn. Cut the head off before the flowers open, but leave the stalk in the ground and it should produce some extra side shoots.

Common problems and how to avoid them

Birds – pigeons love broccoli and other members of the brassica family, and are rarely intimidated by a scarecrow. Covering your plants with netting is likely to be far more effective. Although you could always employ a scarecrow for luck – and a bit of decoration.

Bugs – the cabbage root fly likes to lay its eggs around young broccoli plants leading to destruction by maggots. To prevent this from happening, place 'brassica collars,' or circles of cardboard, around the stems of plants.

The cabbage white butterfly is also a pain. Look out for eggs and brush them off whenever you see them before they develop into great, munching caterpillars. Better still, cover plants with insect-proof netting.

Clubroot – this is a disease that can affect all brassicas, causing the roots to rot. There is no cure and it can survive in the soil for years, so it's important to practice crop rotation and to get rid of any infected plants.

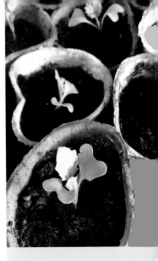

Varieties to try:

Sprouting broccoli
'Claret' – produces lots of purple spears and can tolerate poor soil.

'Late Purple Sprouting' – very hardy with purple spears that can be harvested into spring.

Calabrese varieties
'Belstar' – produces blue-green heads with a good flavour.

'Fiesta' – a reliable variety that can withstand hot summers.

Growing tips

☼ Water regularly, especially during hot weather and keep weeds down by hoeing between plants.

Eat it

BROCCOLI MAKES A great side dish, quickly steamed or stir-fried. For an instant meal, I simply steam it over some pasta, then douse the whole lot in pesto. But don't limit broccoli to the fringe of the plate, it also makes a deserving centre-piece, like this indulgent gratin.

Broccoli and Gorgonzola gratin

Serves 4-6
- **600g broccoli (either sprouting or calabrese)**
- **50g butter**
- **50g plain flour**
- **600ml milk**
- **250g Gorgonzola** (or other blue cheese)
- **2 teaspoons mustard**
- **Black pepper**
- **100g breadcrumbs** (ideally, fresh ones)
- **80g Parmesan, grated**

Method

- Preheat the oven to 190°C/170°C fan/gas 5.

- Steam the broccoli until just tender. It should still have some bite.

- Meanwhile, start making the sauce. Put the butter in a heavy-based saucepan and heat until melted and starting to foam. Stir in the flour and cook for about a minute, or until golden, then add the milk. Keep

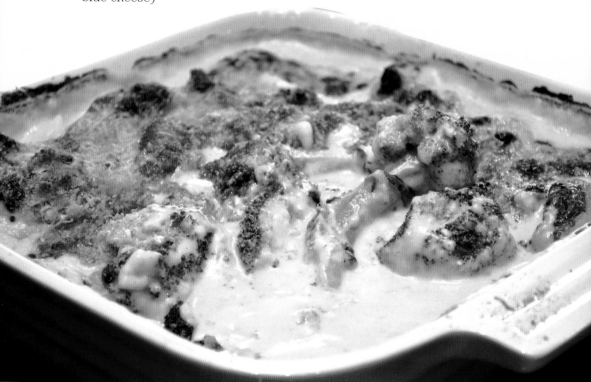

whisking until it starts to simmer and is no longer lumpy. The sauce should thicken as it heats up.

• When the sauce is thick and smooth, remove from the heat. Add the mustard and black pepper and stir in 150g of the Gorgonzola (or other cheese) until it melts.

• Transfer the broccoli to an oven-

proof dish, pour over the sauce and mix thoroughly. Crumble the rest of the blue cheese on top.

• Sprinkle the breadcrumbs and Parmesan over the dish and place in the oven for around 25 minutes or until the top is bubbling and golden.

• Serve with fresh bread and salad leaves.

Very garlicky broccoli

The addition of garlic and oil transforms broccoli from the healthy but ordinary, to the I-can't-believe-this-tastes-so-good-and-it's-still-healthy. Be warned, you may never want to eat unadulterated broccoli again.

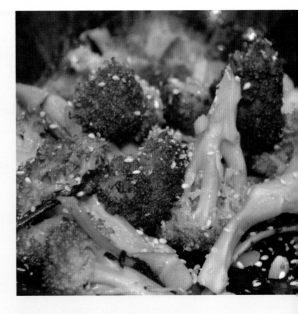

- **A head of broccoli or equivalent amount of spears** (depending on how many people you want to feed)
- **Plenty of garlic, thinly sliced** (around 2 cloves per person, but adapt according to taste)
- **1 tablespoon sesame oil** (or use olive oil if you don't have sesame)
- **Salt**
- **A sprinkling of sesame seeds** (optional)

Method

• Cut the broccoli into florets, or trim the spears if using sprouting broccoli. Steam for a few minutes until half-cooked but still crunchy.

• Meanwhile, heat the oil in a wok. Add the garlic and fry over a medium-low heat for a couple of minutes, being careful not to let it burn. Toss in the broccoli and turn up the heat slightly. Add salt to season and stir fry for a few minutes until just cooked.

• Sprinkle the sesame seeds over the top and serve immediately.

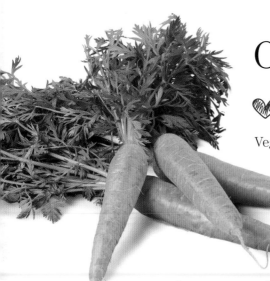

Carrots

♥ Love them

Vegetables don't get much more ubiquitous than carrots, which may explain why they rarely receive much attention. But while they are often regarded as more of a staple than a superfood, the familiar orange roots do have their own super properties. If your grandmother said they would help you see in the dark, she had a point.

Carrots are packed with beta-carotene, an antioxidant, which is converted into vitamin A by the body and is essential for eye health. Beta-carotene is also responsible for the vibrant colour associated with carrots and other orange and yellow fruits and vegetables.

Just one carrot will provide more than twice the amount of Vitamin A needed for one day. Besides helping with vision, vitamin A is also needed for immune function and healthy skin. Studies have also shown that beta-carotene may offer some natural UV protection, helping to defend the skin from sun damage – although consuming large quantities of carrots isn't recommended as an alternative to using sunscreen. And while consuming too much vitamin A can be toxic, the body only converts beta-carotene into as much vitamin A as it needs, making it hard to overdose on carrots – although excessive quantities could cause your skin to turn yellow or orange. Fortunately, this is reversible!

In addition to beta-carotene, carrots also provide vitamins C and K and are a good source of fibre.

Just one carrot will provide more than twice the amount of vitamin A needed for one day ...

✽ Grow them

There is simply no comparison between a shop-bought carrot and one you have grown yourself. Despite their ubiquity, carrots are one of the vegetables that benefit most from being home-grown. Commercially churned out varieties tend to be watery, bizarrely odourless and almost translucent (not to mention laden with pesticides) whereas home-produced ones are densely crunchy and flavoursome. It's like the difference between butter and

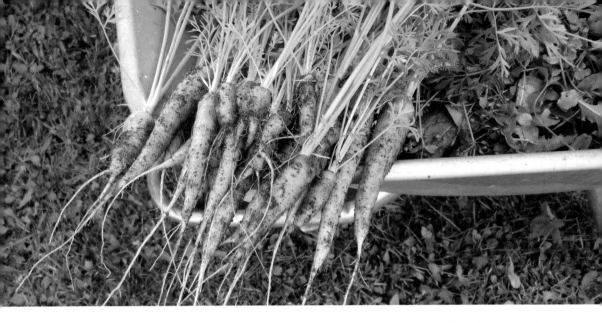

margarine, and only one of those deserves any fridge space.

What's more, while mass produced carrots are unswervingly orange, there's a wide selection of colours to choose from if you grow your own, including: red, yellow, white and even purple. Go crazy and grow a rainbow!

Carrots are one of the vegetables that benefit most from being home-grown ...

Sowing

Carrots are very easy to grow. The main issue is protecting them from carrot fly (see below.)

There are two broad categories of carrots; sweet, summer varieties which can be sown in early spring and picked from May onwards, and maincrop carrots which are sown and harvested later, and will last through the winter if you're lucky.

In March, prepare the soil by digging and raking to break up any lumps. Remove as many stones as you can.

Don't add manure just before sowing, as this will encourage the carrots to fork. Although if they do it's not the end of the world, they just won't win any prizes for looks.

Once the soil is nice and crumbly, create a drill, or narrow channel, in which to sow your seeds. A bamboo cane, or long pole, pressed into the ground does the job for you. Or you can drag a stick, or the end of the rake, along the soil in a straight line.

Water the drills first, then sow the seeds as thinly as possible, ideally leaving about 5cm between each seed. Or you can mix the seed with fine compost or sand before sowing, to help space them out. Leave about 30cms between additional rows. Cover the seeds with fine soil and water gently using a watering can with a rose nozzle so as not to wash the tiny seeds away.

Water occasionally until the seedlings appear, and then only during very dry spells. The weeds will inevitably grow first, but the carrot tops will eventually catch up. Pull the weeds out by hand once the carrots are sturdy enough not to get ripped out in the process. Carrots don't like being disturbed and might respond to any meddling by going a bit floppy, but they will soon recover.

How to combat carrot fly

Enemy number one when it comes to growing carrots is the carrot fly – a tiny insect that can sniff out a carrot from a mile away. It lays its eggs all over the place, and these hatch into maggots that tunnel through the carrots leaving them brown and inedible. Fortunately, there are ways to prevent it from happening in the first place.

Netting

Covering your carrots with insect-proof mesh or netting is by far the best method of keeping your carrots in top condition - or any kind of condition at all. A good way to do this is to make a tunnel using pieces of water pipe bent into semi-circles, or even cheap hula-hoops cut in half, then drape the netting over the frame. Although it can seem like an expense at the time, the netting will last for years and is one of the most worthwhile investments you can make when growing your own food.

The following methods can also be used to deter carrot fly, but these are best used in addition to netting, as an added line of defence:

Companion planting

Plant strong smelling crops like garlic and onions near your carrots as a natural deterrent.

Timing

Pick or thin your carrots on a dull day to minimize the scent which attracts the carrot fly.

Crop rotation

Don't plant carrots in the same spot on consecutive years, as the pupae can stay in the ground over winter and re-emerge in the spring. Though of course, crop rotation won't prevent a new invasion of carrot fly, so this method on its own is unlikely to succeed.

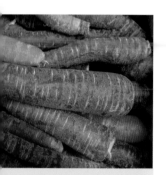

Varieties to try:

'Nantes ' – fast-maturing for early pickings.

'Autumn King' – a popular, heavy cropping maincrop carrot that stores well.

'Purple Haze' – purple skin with orange flesh.

'Parmex' – produces short round-rooted carrots, ideal for growing in containers

'Flyaway' – bred to be resistant to carrot fly.

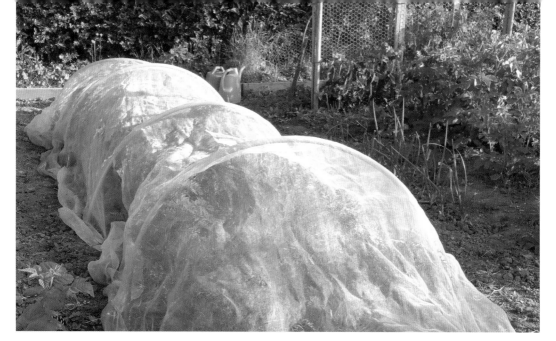

Netting protects from the dreaded carrot fly.

Read the label

If risking a net-free approach, opt for seeds with carrot-fly resistance.

Harvesting and storing carrots

Use a fork or hand fork to dig up carrots. If the soil is very dry, water it first. For winter storage, carrots can be dug up and arranged in layers in boxes (the carrots shouldn't touch each other) and then covered with sand or compost. However, I've always found that carrots will survive in the ground until needed, right through until spring, which saves the time and hassle of having to store them. In cold, frost prone regions, it's advisable to cover the ground with a layer of straw.

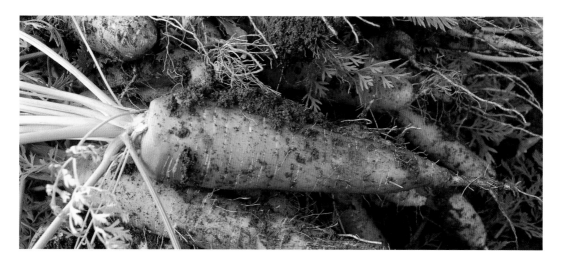

☙ *Eat them*

CARROTS RARELY RECEIVE much love in the kitchen. When short of time or ideas, I often resort to handing them out raw with a pot of hummus, which beats serving them as a soggy, disintegrating heap on the edge of the plate. The nutritional content of carrots is actually enhanced by gentle cooking, but that doesn't mean you need to boil them to oblivion. Forget school dinners, these two recipes provide carrots with a much-needed makeover.

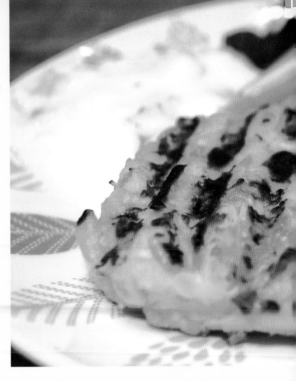

Roasted carrot and butterbean burgers with tzatziki

Cheaper than chips and with very simple ingredients. Roasting the carrots first really brings out the flavour and while they are in the oven you can get on with something else.

Serves 4
- **800g carrots**
- **400g tin of butterbeans, drained**
- **2 small onions**
- **2 eggs, beaten**
- **A splash of rapeseed or olive oil**
- **Salt and pepper to season**

For the tzatziki
- **150g natural yoghurt**
- **4 tablespoons fresh mint, finely chopped**
- **1 tablespoon lemon juice**
- **Half a cucumber, finely diced**
- **1 clove of garlic, crushed** (optional)

Method
- Preheat the oven to 190°C/170°C fan/gas 5.

- Dice the carrot and onion into smallish chunks and place in a roasting dish. Drizzle over the oil and mix so that everything is coated, then season with salt and pepper.

- Place in the oven for around 30 minutes, until the carrots are softened, but not falling apart.

- While the carrots are cooking make the tzatziki by mixing all the ingredients together.

- Remove the carrots from the oven and allow to cool slightly. Add the butterbeans and mash everything together leaving a fairly rough

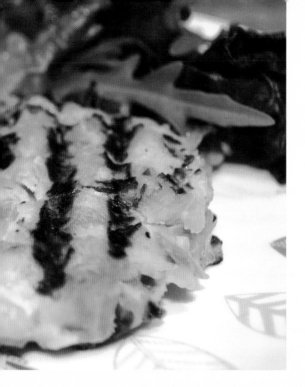

texture. Mix in the beaten egg, then shape into burgers. The mixture can also be made in advance and left in the fridge which firms it up a bit.

• Cook the burgers on a griddle, or in a frying pan, for a few minutes on each side. Serve with the tzatziki, salad and a bun.

Tastes-like-summer carrot salad

A fresh, vibrant salad, without the cloyingness of coleslaw. Don't worry too much about sticking to exact quantities here, just do what works for you.

> **Serves 4-6 as a side dish**
> • **6-8 good sized carrots, coarsely grated or cut into ribbons**
> • **125g sultanas**
> • **50g pine nuts**
> • **2 tablespoons lemon juice**
> • **4 tablespoons olive oil**
> • **A handful of parsley, or coriander, chopped**
> • **Salt and pepper to season**

Method

• Soak the sultanas in hot water for 5 minutes to plump them up, then drain.

• Meanwhile, dry fry the pine nuts over a low heat, stirring all the time until they change colour. Transfer to a plate to cool.

• Combine the carrots, sultanas, lemon juice, olive oil, parsley or coriander, and pine nuts and mix well.

• Season to taste and serve.

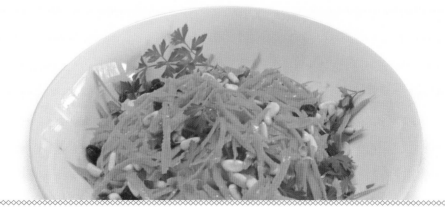

Cauliflower

♥ Love it

Frequently hated by children, and renowned for its rather gassy aroma on cooking, cauliflower is no longer a vegetable to be sniffed at. This vintage veg is enjoying a comeback thanks to its array of health benefits and a new-found versatility in the kitchen.

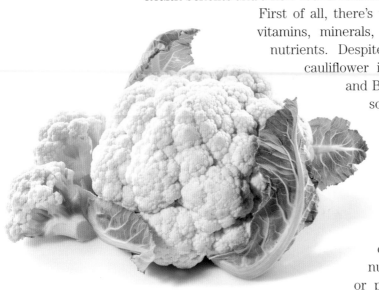

First of all, there's the impressive line-up of vitamins, minerals, antioxidants, and other nutrients. Despite its pallid appearance, cauliflower is rich in vitamins C, K and B vitamins. It's also a good source of manganese, a powerful antioxidant, as well potassium, iron, magnesium and fibre. It even contains some protein and omega-3 fatty acids.

Like its cousin broccoli, cauliflower contains a number of phytochemicals, or plant chemicals, that are thought to protect against cancer and other diseases. These include the compound sulforaphane, which is known for its anticarcinogenic effects. There is plausible evidence that people who regularly eat cauliflower and other brassicas, may be less susceptible to various types of cancer, especially prostate cancer in men. One study found that that men who consumed cauliflower more than once a week were around fifty per cent less likely to be diagnosed with an aggressive form of prostate cancer than those who ate it less than once a month.[27]

> Besides its cancer-fighting properties, cauliflower also contains many anti-inflammatory nutrients ...

Besides its cancer-fighting properties, cauliflower also contains many anti-inflammatory nutrients and these may help with conditions such as arthritis, diabetes, inflammatory bowel disease and ulcerative colitis. So, while there is no such thing as a magic health bullet, regularly eating cauliflower as part of a diet that is rich in fruit and vegetables, may contribute towards a reduced risk of cancer and other diseases.

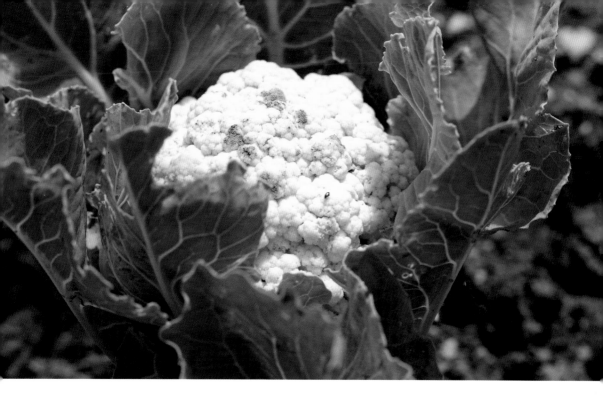

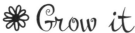 Grow it

Cauliflowers aren't the easiest things to grow, but don't let that put you off. They do require time, attention and regular watering, but that makes them all the more rewarding. There are three types of cauliflower: summer, autumn and winter, so with a bit of planning you can have a year-round supply. This isn't as confusing as it sounds; it's just a case of planting the right variety at the right time of year.

Summer cauliflowers

For the earliest crops, sow seeds indoors in trays or pots in January. Plant the seedlings out in March, and you should have cauliflowers by June.

Autumn (maincrop) cauliflowers

Seed can be sown outdoors, or undercover, in trays or pots in April or May. Transplant seedlings into the ground from May and harvest from August to October.

Winter cauliflowers

Sow seed in pots in May or June, then transplant the seedlings outdoors in August. Leave them in the ground over winter and

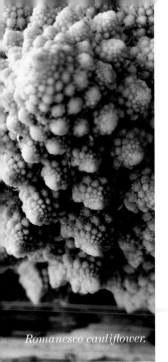

Romanesco cauliflower.

Varieties to try:

'Galleon' – a good quality cauliflower for overwintering , harvest April-May.

'Romanesco' – looks like a cross between cauliflower and broccoli, with beautiful lime green curds and a delicious flavour.

'Igloo' – can be sown close together to produce mini heads, good for small spaces. Sow March-April, harvest July-August.

'Clapton' – bred to be resistant to club root. Harvest in summer and autumn.

harvest from January until spring the following year. If you only grow one type of cauliflower these are a good choice as they require less, if any, watering through the winter, and will be ready to eat when other crops are thin on the ground.

Growing tips

Sow seeds 2cm deep and start them off in pots or trays for the best chance of success.

Transplant seedlings into the ground when they reach a height of 2cm (letting them grow taller can lead to root damage.) Fill the hole with water and let it drain away before dropping the seedling in.

Cauliflowers need lots of space, so unless you are growing a miniature variety, leave 60cm between plants, then press down the soil firmly around the base of the seedling.

Cauliflowers thrive in rich, fertile, firm soil, with an alkaline pH (add lime if necessary) and need regular watering.

Once the white heads appear, fold the surrounding leaves over them and tie them together with string (a hair band also does the trick.) This stops the sun from turning the curds yellow.

Common problems and how to avoid them

Cauliflowers are susceptible to the same problems as other members of the brassica family, including: birds, cabbage root fly, the cabbage white butterfly and clubroot. See the section on broccoli for how to deal with these issues. And at the risk of sounding like a stuck CD, insect-proof netting really is a good investment.

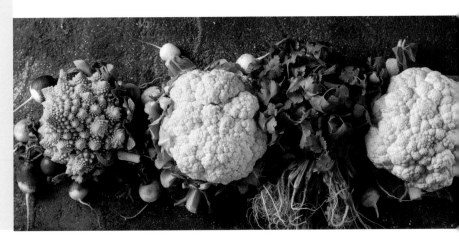

⟨⟩ Eat it

THE ONCE UNLOVED cauliflower is back in fashion and has recently appeared in all sorts of guises; as an alternative to rice, mash and even pizza dough. Although these recent manifestations can be useful if you want to cut back on carbs, cauliflower is at its best when disguised as nothing but itself; steamed, stir-fried, roasted, or covered in cheese sauce. It's also good raw and goes well with a yoghurty, garlicky dip.

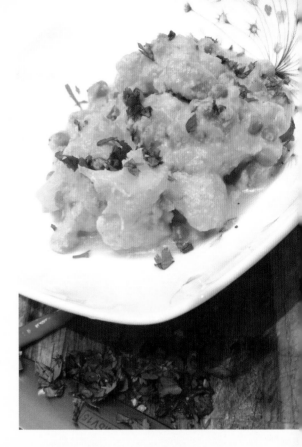

Almond Gobi

This recipe is based on the popular Indian dish, aloo gobi, except this version omits the potato (aloo) leaving more space for the cauliflower (gobi.) The addition of ground almonds gives a deliciously smooth and rich consistency. Gobi is usually eaten as a side dish, but this one shouts main.

Serves 6
- 2 tablespoons rapeseed oil
- 1 large onion, sliced
- 3 carrots, sliced
- 4 cloves of garlic, sliced
- 1 red chilli (less if you don't like heat)
- 4cm piece of fresh ginger, chopped
- 1 teaspoon ground turmeric
- 1½ teaspoons ground cumin
- 1½ teaspoons garam masala

- A pinch or two of salt
- 1 cauliflower, broken into small florets
- 200g peas
- 2 tablespoons sultanas
- 150g ground almonds
- 400ml tin of coconut milk
- A little water
- A handful of coriander, chopped

Method

• Heat the oil in a heavy-based saucepan, and sauté the onion and carrot over a fairly low heat until soft.

• Add the garlic, ginger and chilli and cook for another couple of minutes. Add the dry spices and salt and cook for another five minutes, stirring regularly.

• Add the cauliflower and ground almonds and stir so everything is well coated.

• Add the peas, sultanas, coconut milk and enough water so that everything is just covered.

• Cover and simmer gently for 20-25 minutes, or until the cauliflower is tender.

• Take the lid off and cook quickly on a higher temperature if you need to reduce the liquid.

• Sprinkle with the chopped coriander and serve.

Roasted cauliflower with mustard and chickpeas

Roasting cauliflower instead of boiling or steaming really brings out a new level of nutty sweetness.

Serves 4
- **1 large cauliflower, broken into florets**
- **400g tin chickpeas, drained**
- **2 tablespoons mustard, any kind you like**
- **3 tablespoons olive oil**
- **3 cloves of garlic, crushed**
- **Salt and pepper**

Method

• Preheat the oven to 200°C/180°C fan/gas 6. Line a baking tray with foil.

• Combine the mustard, oil, garlic, salt and pepper in a large bowl. Add the cauliflower and chickpeas and toss until well coated.

• Spread the cauliflower and other ingredients out into a lined baking tray and roast for 25 minutes, turning half way through. The cauliflower is ready when it's tender but not soft.

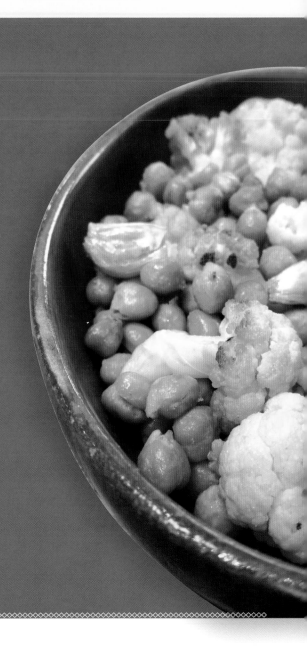

Courgettes

♥ Love them

Courgettes have become the pin-up vegetable of the spiralising movement. But gardeners were advocating them long before people starting making ribbons out of them. Although courgettes, or zucchini as they are also known, aren't as nutrient-dense as some other vegetables, they are certainly a super food in terms of productivity. If you only have time or space to grow a few different crops, then courgettes are worth including for their enthusiasm alone. One plant is capable of churning out an astounding quantity of courgettes and besides giving you plenty to eat, this will make you feel like a seasoned pro in the garden.

And while they don't quite match up to kale on the nutrient chart, courgettes still have plenty of health benefits. They are a very good source of fibre – as long as you don't peel them – and a good source of vitamin C, potassium, magnesium and manganese. They also contain small amounts of other vitamins and minerals.

Another reason to grow courgettes is that you will have a supply of that most elusive of delicacies, the courgette flower. These bright yellow beauties are so fragile that you will rarely, if ever, find them for sale in shops or even markets, which makes them an even more attractive addition to the garden.

> One plant is capable of churning out an astounding quantity of courgettes ...

❀ Grow them

Courgettes are very easy to grow and ridiculously prolific. In the height of summer, a healthy plant can sprout new courgettes seemingly overnight. Just two or three plants are enough to feed a large family – and you will probably end up pleading with the neighbours to take some off your hands, too.

The courgettes you buy in shops tend to be straight and green. But at home, you can grow other varieties too, including yellow ones and round ones. Although these can look impressive, really, the classic ones are the best.

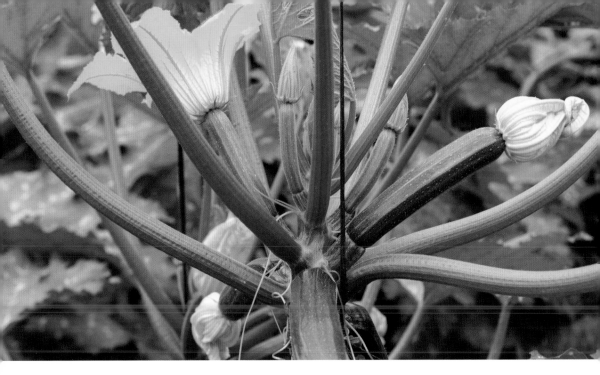

Sowing

In April, sow seeds indoors in large pots of compost at a depth of 2.5cm. Alternatively, you can plant seeds straight outdoors in June, though they will do best with some kind of protection.

Planting out

Courgettes are delicate crops so only plant them outdoors once all risk of frost has passed and it's beginning to feel like summer, usually from late May onwards. Harden the plants off first by placing them outside every day for about a week. Don't forget to bring them in at night, or the drop in temperature will cause them to keel over.

Then choose a warm, bright spot and dig a hole in the ground – courgettes are sun worshippers and will do best in full sun. Turn the pot onto its side and gently tap until the seedling is released with as much of the potting compost around it as possible. Place the seedling in the ground, ideally with some organic matter. Water, refill the hole, then firm the soil down around the plant. Courgettes are bushy plants and can grow quite large, so leave about 90cm around the outside of each plant.

Water daily in dry weather, especially once the plant starts to fruit, and never let the ground dry out.

If space is limited, many varieties of courgette can also be grown in large containers (check the packet first.) Pot-grown plants will require even more watering as the soil will dry out faster.

Pests, problems and how to deal with them

Slugs – although the leaves are slightly prickly this doesn't seem to deter slugs from polishing them off when you're not looking, especially when the plants are very young. So keep the plant in its pot for as long as possible, then transplant it into the ground when it's bigger and less vulnerable. Slugs tend to be less interested in older plants and a larger plant can afford a bit of munching.

For extra protection, cover newly transplanted courgette plants with an upturned transparent container, such as the lid of a propagator or a large plastic bottle cut in half, and keep it in place until the leaves are pressing against the sides. As well as providing a physical barrier against slugs, this also protects the plant from any unexpected changes in the weather.

Powdery mildew – a fungal disease that looks like a dusty substance on the leaves. It can be caused by dry soil, so water regularly to prevent or treat it.

Cucumber Mosaic Virus – leaves will turn yellow and blotchy and the plant will fail. The only cure is to start again.

Harvesting

Pick courgettes when they are small and firm and use a knife to cut them from the plant as they are likely to break if you try to twist or pull them. Courgettes are tastiest when young and regular picking will encourage the plant to keep producing more fruit – not that these plants need much encouragement. Courgettes left on the plant will quickly turn into marrows.

Sexing the courgette

Courgettes have separate male and female flowers (unlike tomatoes for example, whose flowers contain both male and female parts) so rely on pollen being transferred to the female flowers to produce fruit. The best way to ensure this happens is to have a few flowers around to attract pollinating insects (see the earlier section on companion planting.) If necessary, you can pollinate flowers yourself by picking off the male one and rubbing it inside the female one. Or use a paintbrush if you're shy!

Female flowers – have a swelling behind them, which is the start of a little courgette.

Male flowers – have a thin stem behind them and no courgette. These are often the first flowers to be produced.

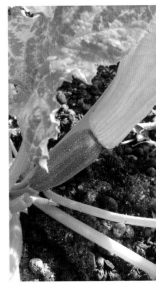

Female flower and courgette.

☙ Eat them

COURGETTES ARE fantastically versatile and can be eaten raw or cooked, and even used in cakes. Due to their high water content, they are best cooked fast and furious without added liquid; sizzled on a barbecue, griddled, fried or stir-fried.

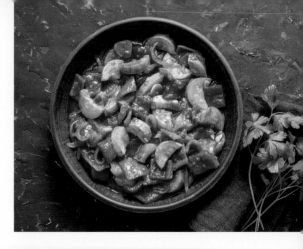

Non-slop ratatouille

Traditional ratatouille is often mushy and swimming in juice. This version has a much more defined texture and taste. The key is to cook all the vegetables separately, so they don't drown each other out. It takes a bit longer, and there's a fair bit of chopping involved, but the end result is worth the extra effort.

Serves 4-6
- **Splash of olive oil**
- **2 red onions, chopped**
- **4 cloves of garlic, finely sliced**
- **2 aubergines**
- **4 courgettes**
- **2 red or yellow peppers**
- **4 large ripe tomatoes**
- **Large sprig of fresh thyme, chopped**
- **1 teaspoon balsamic vinegar**
- **Salt and pepper to season**

Method

- Dice the aubergines, courgettes and peppers into small chunks (around 2cm cubed) but keep each vegetable separate. Set aside.

- Heat a good splash of oil in a large saucepan and sauté the onion with the thyme for a few minutes until soft. Add the garlic and cook for another couple of minutes. Turn off the heat and put the saucepan to one side.

- Heat some oil in a separate frying pan, and fry the aubergine on a fairly high heat, for about 10 minutes, or until browned and softened. Transfer the aubergine to the pan containing the onions.

- Next, fry the courgette on its own, on a high heat so it doesn't become watery, for about 5 minutes, or until browned. Transfer to the large saucepan with the other cooked vegetables.

- Fry the peppers, and add to the mix.

- Skin the tomatoes by scoring a cross in the base of each one with a sharp knife. Then place them in a bowl, cover with boiling water and leave for 30 seconds. Drain, refresh with cold water, then peel the skins away. Dice into chunks.

- Add the diced tomatoes to the rest of the vegetables and place the saucepan back on the heat.

- Add the balsamic vinegar, season, and cook for around 20 minutes.

Money-can't-buy-me fried courgette flowers

If you grow your own courgettes, it would be a crime not to make use of the flowers. By picking the male ones, you won't make a dent in your courgette supply. Or pick the female ones with a mini courgette attached and fry the whole thing. You can cook them plain or stuffed.

- **8 courgette flowers**
  (or as many as you have available)
- **Plenty of sunflower oil for frying**

For the batter
- **100g self-raising flour**
- **150ml ice-cold, sparkling water**
- **Pinch of salt**

For the filling (optional)
- **200g goat's cheese**
- **Sprig of thyme, leaves finely chopped**

Method

• If possible, pick the flowers when you are ready to use them and when they are open. Don't wash them, but check there aren't any insects hiding inside.

• To make the batter, combine the flour and salt, then whisk in the water until smooth. It should be quite runny, so add more water if necessary.

• For the filling (if using), mix together the goat's cheese and thyme. Then spoon some into each

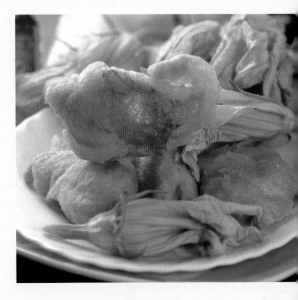

flower. Twist the petals together at the top to cover the filling.

• Pour the sunflower oil into a large, heavy-based saucepan so that it's about one third full. The oil is hot enough when a breadcrumb dropped inside, sizzles and turns brown. When it reaches this point, take a flower (with the filling inside, if using) and quickly dip it into the batter. Shake off the excess, then carefully lower the flower into the oil and cook for around two minutes until crisp and golden.

• Remove with a slotted spoon and place on some kitchen paper to absorb the excess oil. Cook all the flowers this way, but no more than two or three at a time or the temperature of the oil will drop.

• Season with salt and serve immediately. And enjoy in the knowledge that this is a dish money can't buy.

French Beans

♥ Love them

Crunchy, vibrant and prolific, French beans are one of the most rewarding crops you can grow at home, producing bumper pickings throughout the summer and into autumn.

Supermarkets tend to sell only the generic, slender, green varieties, but French beans appear in a multitude of shapes, sizes, and colours, including purple, yellow and speckled. And unlike their runner bean cousins, there's none of that dental-floss stringiness. The dainty pods contain a cocktail of fibre, protein, vitamins, minerals and antioxidants. Like other beans, they provide a decent supply of vitamins A, C and K. They are also a good source of folate, iron, calcium, magnesium, copper, manganese and potassium. French beans also contain substantial amounts of phenolic acids and flavonoids and these powerful antioxidants may help stave off many serious illnesses.[28]

Studies have pointed to a link between the consumption of beans and a lowered risk of various cancers and heart disease. And if you can get hold of speckled varieties, these have been shown to have the highest antioxidant levels of all.[29] Beans may also act as an anti-diabetes and weight-loss food as they are digested slowly, helping to stabilise blood sugar and promote a feeling of fullness, which makes these attractive crops an all-round nutritional winner.

Beans may also act as an anti-diabetes and weight-loss food as they are digested slowly ...

❋ Grow them

There are two main types of French beans: dwarf and climbing. Both are easy to grow, but for sheer quantity the climbing ones are best.

French beans are tender crops, so don't tolerate the cold. For this reason, they are usually started off in pots indoors in April, before being planted outdoors in May or early June.

Fill small pots with damp potting compost and place a single seed 5cm deep into each pot. Cover with a little more compost and leave on a warm windowsill to germinate. When the seedlings are about 10cm tall, harden them off by leaving the pots outside for a few hours each day, bringing them in again at night. Do this for about a week, gradually increasing the time they spend outside each day to get them acclimatised to the outdoors. When all chance of frost has passed, transplant the seedlings into the ground, leaving about 15cm between plants.

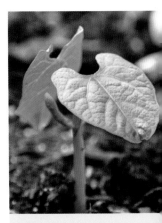

Although starting French beans off indoors is the most failproof method, you can save time and effort by sowing them directly into the ground from late May, especially in warmer regions. Sow two seeds together, then remove the weaker one if both germinate.

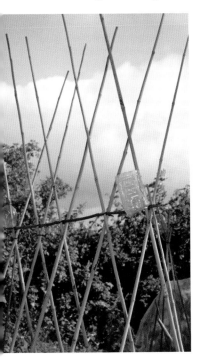

As the name suggests, climbing varieties of French beans need something to climb up as they grow. Bamboo canes work well, either in a tepee formation, or with two rows of canes sloping towards each other so the tops cross over. For better stability and wind resistance, cross the canes lower down rather than near the top, so they form an 'x' shape. As the beans grow they will wrap themselves around the canes, but if they struggle to get a grip early on, help them out with plant ties or string.

Once the plants reach the top of the canes, pinch out the growing tip to encourage the growth of side shoots and more beans. Keep the plants well-watered, especially during dry periods and when they are in flower.

Dwarf beans grow into low bushes, so shouldn't need support to help them stand up.

Harvest

The first beans should be ready to eat about two months after planting. The more you pick, the more will grow, so harvest regularly. The first beans to appear will be low down the plant close to the ground, so don't forget to check – it's easy to miss them.

Top tips

☀ When planting beans directly outside, place an upturned jam jar or half a plastic bottle over the soil where the bean has been sown, to provide extra warmth and protection from slugs.

☀ Wrap some bubble wrap loosely around newly transplanted seedlings in case of a drop in temperature.

☀ Sow new seeds every 3 weeks until August for a continuous crop into October.

☀ Always sow a few extra seeds in case any fail to germinate or fall prey to pests.

☀ Plant marigolds next to beans to deter aphids.

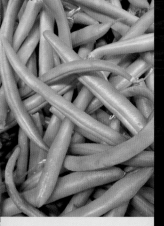

Varieties to try:

'Cobra' – reliable and prolific with lovely, tender pods. A climbing variety.

'Blue Lake' – a popular climbing variety that produces heaps of tender, tasty pods.

'Purple Teepee' – a dwarf type that produces pretty purple pods that turn green on cooking.

'Sprite' – a very compact dwarf variety that produces delicious straight beans.

'Barlotta Lingua Di Fuoco' – Italian climbing French bean whose names translates as 'Tongues of Fire'. It produces attractive red, purple and green speckled pods that can be eaten young, or allowed to mature into haricot beans.

ᗜ Eat them

SOMETIMES, SIMPLE IS best. Freshly picked French beans need little more than a decent dressing to make them shine. This one takes just minutes to prepare.

French beans with lemon and garlic

Serves 4 as a side dish
- **350g French beans**
- **1 tablespoon lemon juice**
- **1 tablespoon finely grated lemon zest**
- **3 tablespoons olive oil**
- **1 clove of garlic, crushed**
- **Salt and pepper**

Method

• Make the dressing by putting the lemon zest and juice, olive oil, garlic and seasoning in a jar. Put the lid on tightly and give it all a good shake.

• Bring a pan of salted water to the boil. Drop the beans into the water and cook for 2 or 3 minutes. They should turn bright green, but retain some crunch.

• Transfer the beans to a bowl and pour the dressing over while they are still warm.

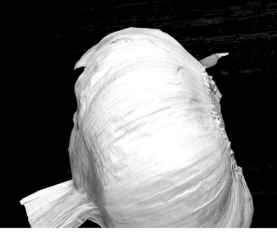

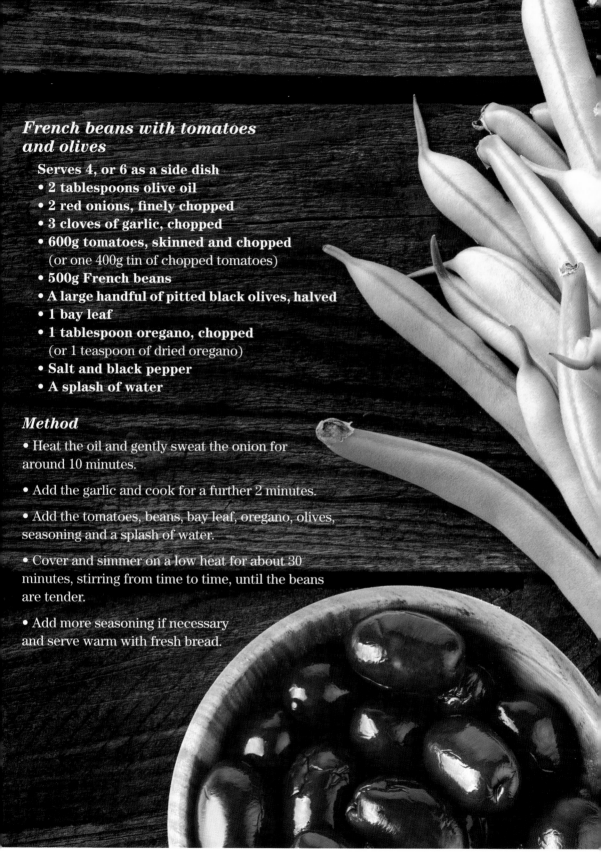

French beans with tomatoes and olives

Serves 4, or 6 as a side dish
- 2 tablespoons olive oil
- 2 red onions, finely chopped
- 3 cloves of garlic, chopped
- 600g tomatoes, skinned and chopped
  (or one 400g tin of chopped tomatoes)
- 500g French beans
- A large handful of pitted black olives, halved
- 1 bay leaf
- 1 tablespoon oregano, chopped
  (or 1 teaspoon of dried oregano)
- Salt and black pepper
- A splash of water

Method

• Heat the oil and gently sweat the onion for around 10 minutes.

• Add the garlic and cook for a further 2 minutes.

• Add the tomatoes, beans, bay leaf, oregano, olives, seasoning and a splash of water.

• Cover and simmer on a low heat for about 30 minutes, stirring from time to time, until the beans are tender.

• Add more seasoning if necessary and serve warm with fresh bread.

Florence Fennel

♥ Love it

Not to be confused with the herb that shares its name, Florence Fennel is prized for the deliciously crisp and aromatic bulbs that bulge from the ground beneath a shower of feathery green foliage. The closely related herb on the other hand is grown mainly for its leaves and seeds.

A favourite in Italy, Florence fennel, or fennel as it's usually known, is less familiar in the UK and is likely to mystify gardeners and cooks alike – although cooking is by no means essential; it's perfect for eating raw, too.

Fennel has been part of traditional medicine for centuries and you can practically taste its soothing, cleansing powers with each aniseedy bite. This uniquely-flavoured vegetable is a natural anti-inflammatory and is used to alleviate stomach aches, indigestion, bloating, flatulence and irritable bowel syndrome. In some cultures, the seeds are chewed after meals to aid digestion and get rid of bad breath. They can also be steeped in boiling water to make a stomach-calming tea.

There is something inherently feminine about fennel, too. Perhaps the smooth curves, or the fact that it has been shown to help reduce menstrual pain and bleeding[30] and even lessen the severity of premenstrual syndrome.[31] The potent ingredient is an essential oil called anethole. Besides reducing inflammation, this natural compound has antibacterial and anti-fungal properties and contributes to the plant's carminative (anti-flatulent) effects.

Fennel may also help calm colicky babies – and their frazzled parents. One study found that infants treated with fennel seed oil were reported to have sixty-five per cent less colic, measured by crying episodes, than those given a placebo.[32] As miraculous as this sounds, there is still no established safe way to treat babies with fennel, so the safest option is for breastfeeding mothers to drink fennel tea, which is thought to have the added bonus of increasing milk flow. Fortunately, with or without fennel, colic doesn't last forever!

In addition to its healing properties, fennel is high in fibre and rich in vitamin C. This supercharged vegetable also contains many

This uniquely-flavoured vegetable is a natural anti-inflammatory and is used to alleviate stomach aches, indigestion, bloating, flatulence and irritable bowel syndrome ...

important minerals including: potassium, iron, calcium, copper, zinc, and selenium. With a refreshing taste to boot, it could be just your cup of (fennel) tea.

✿ Grow it

The blunt truth is that Florence fennel is a challenging vegetable to grow, at least in the UK. But nothing ventured, nothing gained. The worst that can happen is you end up a load of foliage and no bulb. For years, this was all I achieved and although the greenery was edible, it was scant consolation for the lack of anything more substantial.

You can save yourself the same disappointment by sticking to one rule; don't plant fennel until June! Although this seems ridiculously late, especially when your other seeds have turned into an army of teenage seedlings, delaying planting seems to be the best route to success with fennel. This is a plant that needs light and warmth, and has the patience of a toddler if it doesn't get it.

Sowing

Fennel doesn't like being transplanted so it's best sown straight into the ground in mid-June. Sow the seed thinly into drills that are 1cm deep and water gently. Once the seedlings are established, thin them out to leave gaps of 30cm between plants.

Aftercare

Fennel is notorious for bolting, or turning to seed before it has produced a bulb. This happens if it's too cold or too dry, so regular watering is critical. It also helps to mulch around the plants to conserve moisture. And if you can give it an organic feed like liquid seaweed every couple of weeks, even better.

As the bulbs swell, build up the earth around them to increase the size and quality. Harvest them once they reach tennis ball-size. This should be around mid-October for seed sown in the middle of June.

Problems

The good news is pests and diseases don't tend to bother with fennel, so all you need to worry about is the weather and there's not an awful lot you can do about that, although to improve your chances of success, opt for bulbs that are bred to be resistant to bolting.

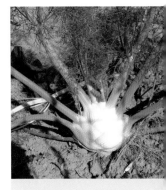

Varieties to try:

'**Perfection**' – larger than average bulbs with a delicate flavour. Bolting resistant.

'**Cantino**' – sweet tasting bulbs with a refreshing aniseed flavour. Bolting resistant.

'**Amigo**' – uniform, slightly flattened bulbs. Very resistant to bolting.

'**Colossal**' – large, bolt-resistant bulbs.

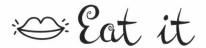

Eat it

THE SIMPLEST WAY to enjoy
Florence fennel is to chop the stalks
away from the bulb, then cut it down
the middle into sections and eat raw,
dipped in olive oil and balsamic vinegar.
Placing the cut segments in a bowl
of cold water helps keep them crisp.
Fennel can also be grated or chopped
and used in salads. For something more
adventurous, try this Italian-inspired
dish with cheese and walnuts.

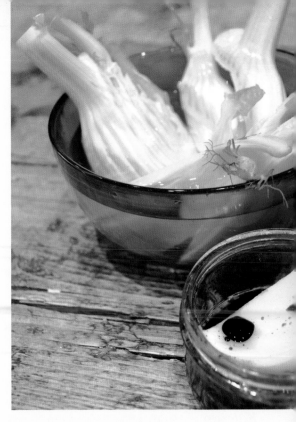

Oven roasted fennel with walnuts

Serves 4
- **4 large fennel bulbs**
- **100g Gouda cheese**
  (or Fontina if you can get it.)
- **100g Parmesan, grated**
- **A little butter for greasing**
- **80g walnuts, roughly chopped**
- **10g wholemeal flour**
- **A sprinkling of grated nutmeg**
- **Salt and pepper**

Method

- Preheat the oven to 180°C /160°C
fan/gas 4.

- Chop the fennel into large chunks
and place in boiling, salted water for
around 10 minutes.

- Remove the fennel from the water
and pat dry.

- Use the butter to grease a large oven-
proof dish, then sprinkle with flour.

- Arrange the fennel in the dish,
then dot with the Gouda (or
Fontina) and walnuts. Add a pinch of

salt and pepper and sprinkle
the Parmesan and nutmeg
over the top.

- Bake for 15 minutes until
bubbling and golden.

Easy fennel and fish tagine with couscous

Serves 4
- **Oil for frying**
- **500g of firm white fish,
  eg hake or monkfish, cut into cubes**
- **2 red onions, finely chopped**
- **4 cloves of garlic, crushed**
- **1 red chilli, deseeded and
  finely chopped**
  (use less for a milder flavour)
- **1.5cm root ginger, finely chopped**
- **1 teaspoon ground cumin**

- **2x 400g tins chopped tomatoes**
- **600ml fish or vegetable stock**
- **2 bulbs of fennel, thinly sliced**
- **Large handful of fresh coriander, roughly chopped**
- **200g couscous (or bulgur wheat)**
- **400ml boiling water**
- **80g green olives, roughly chopped**
- **Good squeeze of lemon juice**

Method

• To prepare the couscous, place it in a large bowl and pour over 400ml of boiling water and a squeeze of lemon juice. (If using bulgur wheat, prepare according to the instructions on the packet.) Cover and leave to stand.

• Meanwhile, heat the oil in a large frying pan. Add the onion and cook for 5 minutes, until soft. Add the garlic, ginger, chilli and spices and cook for another 3 minutes. Pour in the tomatoes and stock and simmer for 5 minutes.

• Add the fennel and simmer for another 10 minutes, until tender. Add the fish and half the coriander and cook gently for around 5-10 minutes, or until the fish is cooked through.

• Season if necessary.

• Fluff up the couscous (or bulgur wheat) with a fork, then stir in the olives and the rest of the coriander and serve with the tagine.

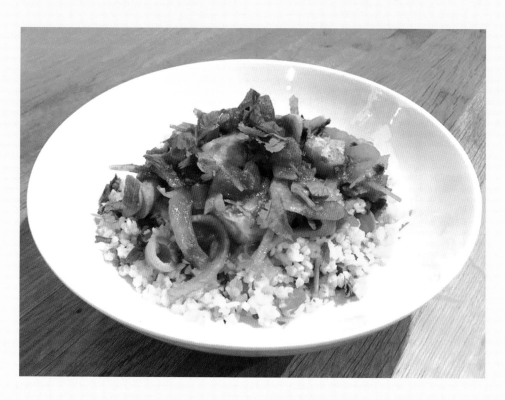

Garlic

♥ Love it

From vampire deterrent to aphrodisiac, medicine to superfood, garlic has been prized throughout the ages for its healing properties as well as its culinary strength. It was used by the Romans and Egyptians and other ancient civilisations, and is widely mentioned in the Ebers Papyrus, one of the oldest medicinal texts.

This small but potent vegetable is a natural antibiotic and was known as 'Russian Penicillin' during the two world wars. It also has anti-fungal and anti-viral properties and has been used for centuries to treat a miscellany of conditions from tummy bugs to toothache, warts to arthritis. It was even thought to ward off the plague.

Folklore aside, garlic provides an excellent source of vitamin B6, vitamin C and many minerals including: manganese, selenium, phosphorous, calcium, potassium, iron and copper. But its star property appears to be the sulphur compound, allicin. This is formed when garlic is crushed or chopped, giving rise to that unmistakable aroma. Once released, allicin rapidly breaks down to form a number of other compounds, which have been the subject of much research. Numerous studies have shown that garlic can reduce both high cholesterol levels and high blood pressure.[33,34] This could have important implications for cardiovascular disease – the leading killer worldwide.

There is a also a wealth of information on garlic's cancer-fighting potential, with evidence that increased garlic consumption may reduce the risk of various cancers, especially those of the stomach, colon and bowel, oesophagus, pancreas, breast and lung.[35] Tests have also shown that garlic can kill the Helicobacter pylori. This is the most common bacterial infection in the world and can live in the digestive tract and sometimes lead to stomach ulcers and gastric cancer.[36]

Garlic may help protect against lung cancer, too. One large study found that adults who ate raw garlic at least twice a week were 44

Numerous studies have shown that garlic can reduce both high cholesterol levels and high blood pressure ...

per cent less likely to develop the disease. Even when smoking was taken into consideration, garlic was still found to reduce the risk by around 30 per cent.[37]

Of course, no 'superfood' can compensate for an unhealthy lifestyle – or even a healthy one. But as one of the most widely researched medicinal plants on earth, there's a good case that garlic's potency may stretch well beyond the kitchen. However, as the therapeutic powers are impaired or destroyed by cooking, garlic is best eaten raw. A temporary bout of bad breath could be a small price (for others) to pay for the potential health benefits.

❋ Grow it

Garlic is one of the easiest crops of all to grow. Simply split the bulb into individual cloves and push each clove into the soil, flat end first until the tip is just below the soil surface. Leave it alone for a few months, and hey presto, each clove will have photocopied itself into a whole new bulb.

There are two types of garlic: hard-neck and soft-neck. Hard-neck types have large cloves and a strong flavour but don't keep as well as soft-necks. Soft-necks are the ones likely to be sold in

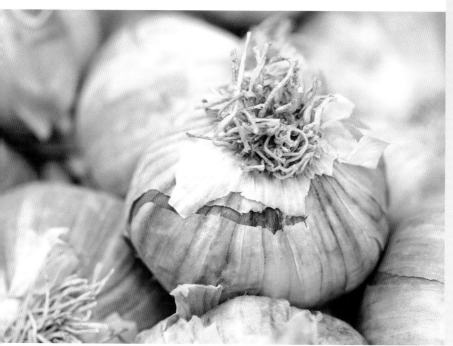

Varieties to try:

'Sultop' – easy to peel flavoursome cloves. This variety is more suited to spring than autumn planting. A hard-neck variety.

'Purple White' – produces purple striped bulbs with strong tasting cloves. A hard-neck variety.

'Cristo' – a classic French soft-neck variety with white skin, pinkish flesh and good flavour. Stores well.

'Elephant' – as the name suggests, this variety produces huge bulbs. Technically, it's actually a leek, but is grown in the same way as garlic and has a mild flavour.

'Romanian Red' – with one of the highest concentrations of allicin of all garlic varieties, this one can be hard to get hold of. It produces very large cloves, sometimes only four per bulb, with a strong flavour. A hard-neck variety.

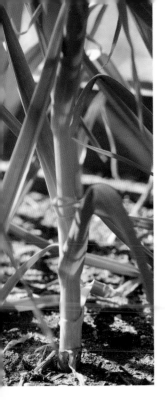

Once lifted, spread the bulbs out somewhere warm to dry before storing ...

shops, having been imported, and can be stored for longer. They have bendy stems that can be plaited.

How to plant

• The best time to plant garlic is during October or November, as it needs a cold spell to encourage strong growth. If you miss this window, it can also be planted in February or March, but the bulbs will be smaller.

• Choose a sunny position, and avoid planting in waterlogged soil. If your soil is very wet and heavy, try adding some grit and sand to the hole before planting.

• Leave about 15cm between each clove and 25cm between rows.

• Don't bother trying to plant supermarket garlic, which may harbour diseases, and has probably been bred for a different climate.

• Weed regularly as garlic doesn't like competition and only water during very dry spells. Over watering can cause the bulbs to rot.

• Garlic tends to be fairly trouble-free, but as with all crops avoid planting garlic in the same spot in consecutive years, to prevent diseases building up.

• If the birds try to dig it up, cover with chicken wire or netting for the first few weeks.

Harvesting

Garlic planted in autumn will be ready to harvest in June and July. Varieties planted in spring will be ready a bit later.

The bulbs are ready to dig up once the leaves turn yellow and floppy. Loosen them from the soil with a fork, being careful not to pierce them, then gently pull them up.

Don't leave garlic in the soil for too long after the foliage has turned yellow, as this can cause the bulbs to sprout again and then rot in storage. And never water after this stage.

If you want green garlic (young garlic) just dig it up earlier. This will have a milder flavour and creamier texture.

⌣ Eat it

I RARELY COOK anything without garlic, except desserts that is – although I have heard of it used in cakes, ice-cream and even beer. I think I'll pass on those. If you have never eaten raw garlic, then this bruschetta is the perfect introduction.

Extra strong bruschetta

The raw garlic in this recipe preserves the health benefits of the allicin – and gives it an extra kick.

- **Plenty of ripe tomatoes**
- **2 or 3 cloves of garlic – more if you dare**
- **A loaf of ciabatta, or other bread, sliced**
- **A splash of olive oil**
- **A shake of oregano**
- **Salt and pepper**

Method

• Crush one or two cloves of garlic, reserving at least one whole clove.

• Dice the tomatoes and place in a bowl with a glug of olive oil, the oregano, salt, pepper and crushed garlic. Mix well.

• Toast the bread under the grill, or on a barbecue.

• Cut the remaining garlic clove in half, then rub the cut surface all over the toasted bread.

• Spoon some of the diced tomato mixture onto the toasted bread and serve.

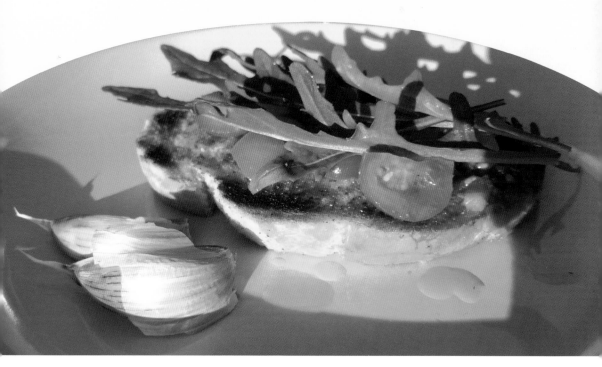

Garlic, courgette and pesto soup

Bursting with freshness and flavour, this soup is unlike anything you will ever find in a tin, or even a carton. The garlic is added raw to minimise cooking and maximise the health benefits, but for a milder flavour, just fry it with the courgette at the start. This recipe is also a fantastic way of using up home-grown courgettes, which invariably produce a summer glut if you grow your own.

Serves 4
- **4 cloves of garlic, finely chopped** (vary the amount according to taste)
- **5 medium courgettes**
- **3 tablespoons pesto**
- **Salt and pepper**
- **750ml chicken or vegetable stock**
- **Handful of parsley, chopped**
- **Glug of olive oil**

Method

- Cut the courgettes in half lengthways, then chop into thin half-moon shaped slices.

- Heat the oil, then add the courgette, season with salt and pepper and fry on a fairly high heat for 10-15 minutes, until the courgettes are a rich golden colour. (Add the garlic at this stage too if you don't want the flavour to be too strong).

- Add the pesto, mix well, and fry for another couple of minutes. Add the stock and simmer for 10 minutes. Allow to cool slightly.

- Add the garlic (if you didn't add it before) and parsley, blend everything together and serve.

Kale

♥ Love it

If there is one food that has come
to symbolise the whole 'superfood'
movement, it's kale. Despite the
hype, it is in fact ridiculously good
for you, containing an almost
unrivalled line up of vitamins,
minerals and nutrients. The dark green
leaves are packed with vitamins A, C and K. Just
one portion of kale supplies more than your daily needs
(RNI) of all these vitamins. Raw kale contains more than
double the amount of vitamin C found in the same weight of
oranges, and even cooked kale still comes out on top[16].

Kale is also exceptionally high in vitamin K which plays a
key role in blood clotting and healthy bones and may protect
against osteoarthritis. This celebrated brassica is rich in many
vital minerals too, like iron and calcium, as well as antioxidants
including lutein, a carotenoid that is essential for eye health.

To add to these already impressive credentials, kale is also full
of a group of compounds known as glucosinolates. These sulphur-
containing chemicals are broken down during food preparation
and consumption to form other potent compounds such as indoles
and isothiocyanates which have been shown to have anti-cancer
effects.

Although research is ongoing, these substances may help
eliminate carcinogens from the body before they damage DNA,
making kale a potentially important weapon in helping to prevent,
and combat, various types of cancer.

> Raw kale contains
> more than double the
> amount of vitamin
> C found in the same
> weight of oranges ...

❊ Grow it

Don't be put off by the fact it's a brassica. Kale is gratifyingly easy
to grow and much less fussy than most of its cousins. It will put up
with most soil types and doesn't mind a bit of neglect.

There are two main types of kale: flat-leaved, and the more
common curly-leaved varieties.

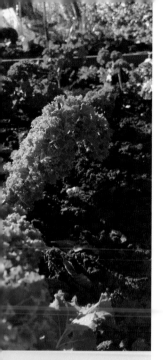

Varieties to try:

'Dwarf Green Curled' – produces attractive, dark, tightly frilled leaves.

'Pentland Brig' – an old-fashioned variety with less curly leaves.

'Red Russian' – pretty grey-green leaves with purple veins. Can be planted close together for a continuous supply of young leaves which are good in salads.

'Cavolo Nero' – also known as 'Tuscan kale' or 'Black Kale,' has long, slender, dark coloured leaves with a slightly sweet flavour.

Seeds can be sown in pots indoors in March, or outdoors from April, either in trays or a temporary seed bed. Plant seeds at a depth of 1cm.

Seven or eight weeks later, or once your seedlings have five or six leaves, you can transplant them to their final growing positions.

Seedlings raised indoors will need to be hardened off first, so leave the pots outdoors for a few hours each day over the course of a week, to get them used to the change in temperature.

Like most crops, kale does best in a sunny spot, but a bit of shade is okay if that's all you have.

It makes sense to grow kale as a cut-and-come again crop, as this provides a continuous supply of young leaves. Or you can leave the plants to mature for a source of winter greens.

For cut and come again leaves, seedlings can be planted close together, with as little as 10cm between them. If you're planning to let the plants reach their full size, then space them 45cm apart.

Before planting each seedling, dig a hole, fill it with water a couple of times, and let the water drain into the ground. This will encourage the roots to work their way down and reduce the need for watering later on. Position the seedling inside the hole so that the lowest leaves are level with the ground, then press down the soil around the base of the plant.

Once in the ground, kale plants are surprisingly self-sufficient. Simply water every 10-14 days during dry spells and weed when you have a few spare minutes. It's a good idea to cover the plants with netting to keep butterflies away. Alternatively, pick the caterpillars off when they emerge – preferably before they reach your plate. Netting also stops birds, and particularly pigeons, from attacking the crops.

Harvesting

From early November, start picking the leaves. They key is to pick little and often and always cut from the crown or top to encourage more leaves to grow. Side shoots will form from February.

There's no need to worry about cold – kale can survive temperatures as a low as minus 15 degrees and frost actually improves the flavour, by helping turn the starches into sugar. With any luck, it should keep going until May, making kale an ideal crop for bridging the hungry gap between winter and spring, when there's pitifully little else available.

✑ Eat it

KALE HAS BECOME synonymous with clean-eating and green smoothies. If you genuinely enjoy drinking liquidised brassicas for breakfast, then brilliant, go for it. If on the other hand you have to gulp it down with your nose held, then stick to something else like porridge, or eggs in the morning and save the kale for later. Healthy food should never be gruelling – that only makes the bad stuff seem more appealing. When good food tastes good, the collateral benefits will follow.

Fortunately, there are plenty of tasty ways to reap the nutritional rewards of kale. Although it's passable steamed and served as a side dish, this is a vegetable that does best with company. Add it to soups, salads, pasta dishes and stir fries. Or for a real crowd-pleaser turn it into healthy crisps.

Kale crisps

These might not bear much resemblance to a packet of ready salted, but they will do you a lot more good. They are also good for winning over kale-sceptics and children.

- **A few handfuls of kale**
- **1 tablespoon rapeseed or olive oil**
- **Salt**
- **Smoked paprika**
  (or any other seasoning that takes your fancy like cajun spices, chilli or cumin.)

Method

• Preheat the oven to 150°C/130°C fan/gas 2.

• Tear the kale into small strips, discarding the stalks. Wash and dry.

• Place in a bowl and massage with the oil and seasoning.

• Place the shiny strips of kale in a single layer on a baking tray. Don't be tempted to pile them up or they will go soggy – cook in batches instead.

• Bake for 15 - 20 minutes, keeping a close eye so that they don't burn, then remove from the oven and leave to cool. The kale will go more crispy as it cools.

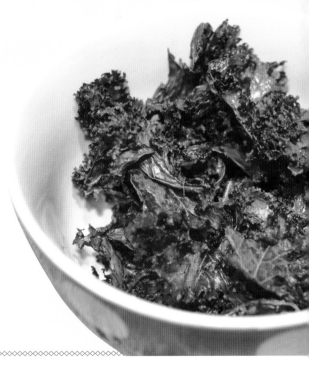

Stir-fried kale with cashew nuts

It's hard to imagine a healthier meal than this. Throw in some meat, prawns, or tofu if you like.

Serves 4
- **700g kale, stalks and central veins removed, torn into small pieces**
- **2 tablespoons rapeseed oil**
- **1 onion, chopped**
- **4 cloves of garlic, chopped**
- **1 small red chilli, finely chopped** (optional)
- **2 carrots, cut into very thin strips**
- **1 red pepper, thinly sliced**
- **1 yellow pepper, thinly sliced**
- **150g broccoli, divided into small florets**
- **150g beansprouts**
- **4-5 tablespoons vegetable stock**
- **2 tablespoons soy sauce**
- **A generous handful of cashew nuts**

Method

• Heat the oil in a pre-heated wok. Add the onion and stir-fry for about 3 minutes.

• Throw in the garlic, carrot, broccoli, chilli (if using) and peppers and stir-fry for a few more minutes until the peppers are tender.

• Add the kale and stir fry for another couple of minutes.

• Pour in the stock, reduce the heat and simmer for a few minutes until the kale is soft. Add the beansprouts and soy sauce, cook for a further 2 minutes, then stir in the nuts.

• Serve with rice or noodles.

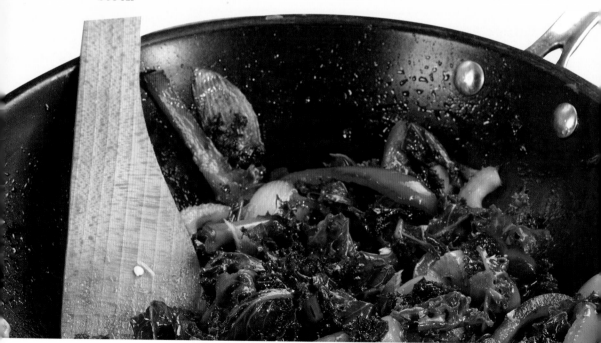

Kohlrabi

💚 Love it

This extraordinary looking vegetable, resembling a cross between a turnip and a UFO, is still trying to nudge its way out of obscurity. Despite a few attempts to tout it as 'superfood,' kohlrabi is rarely sold in the UK, although it is popular in Germany and parts of Eastern Europe.

Regardless of its status – or lack of – kohlrabi is extremely good for you. It provides a super source of vitamin C – not quite as much as that notorious over-achiever kale, but still more than oranges. It's also rich in potassium. Like other brassicas, kohlrabi contains phytochemicals, or plant chemicals, that are believed to have anti-cancer and anti-inflammatory effects. It's also high in fibre, very low in calories, and a good source of minerals including: copper, manganese, iron, and calcium.

With its combination of nutritional benefits and a mild, crisp taste it's hard to see what's not to like about kohlrabi – except the fact you can rarely get hold of it. All the more reason to grow it yourself, then.

✳ Grow it

Don't be fooled by the exotic appearance. Kohlrabi doesn't need an exotic climate in which to grow, and copes well with cool conditions.

It's almost worth growing for its ornamental value alone. The bulbous stem with its antennae-like shoots is strangely beautiful and is a good choice if you want to spice up your plot with a few unusual specimens, or impress your friends.

Better still, kohlrabi is fairly low maintenance and doesn't hog loads of space. Some varieties can even be raised in containers. It's very quick to mature and can be ready to eat just sixty days after planting – not exactly fast food, but still good for impatient gardeners. It's also ideal for intercropping. This is where crops

> Like other brassicas, kohlrabi contains phytochemicals, or plant chemicals, that are believed to have anti-cancer and anti-inflammatory effects ...

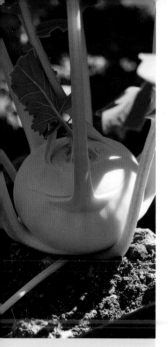

Varieties to try:

'Kongo' – high quality and fast maturing. Pale green with sweet, juicy flesh.

'Superschmelz' – a giant variety with green skin and white flesh. The bulbs can reach an impressive 25cm in diameter, while remaining sweet and tender.

'Azur Star' – violet bulbs that are resistant to bolting.

'Kohlribi' – a purple skinned variety that stays sweet and juicy when other varieties are past their best. Good for a late harvest.

that are quick to mature are planted in between those that like to take their time, to maximise available ground space. So slot a few kohlrabi among long-haul brassicas like kale or Brussels sprouts, and pick them while their larger, slower relatives are still growing.

Sowing

There are two main types of kohlrabi: pale green and and purple. The green ones are faster growing, and can be planted from early spring onwards. Purple varieties are hardier and can be sown from mid-summer for autumn and winter pickings.

For the earliest crops, start seed off indoors in February or March and transplant the seedlings outdoors when they reach 5cm.

Or for an easier, lazier option, wait until April, then scatter the seed directly outside. Sow thinly at a depth of 1.5cm and cover over with soil. Leave 30cm between rows and thin seedlings out before they become too big, leaving gaps of around 20cm between plants, depending on the variety. Or grow them closer together for miniature veg.

An alkaline soil is best, so add some lime if necessary, or grow in pots of compost if you have very acidic soil.

Aftercare

Water regularly to prevent the bulbs from becoming woody, and keep the soil weed free. Adding a layer of organic mulch will help and will also improve the soil.

For a continuous crop, plant new seeds every few weeks until August, and harvest until December.

Kohlrabi is best eaten young, so start harvesting the bulbs once they reach golf ball size, and don't let them become larger than a tennis ball (unless you are growing a giant variety.) It doesn't store brilliantly once picked, so is best eaten fresh.

Problems and troubleshooting

Kohlrabi is easier to grow than many other brassicas, and less susceptible to pests and diseases. However, pigeons, club-root and cabbage root-fly can all present a problem. (See the section on broccoli for dealing with and avoiding these.)

✧ Eat it

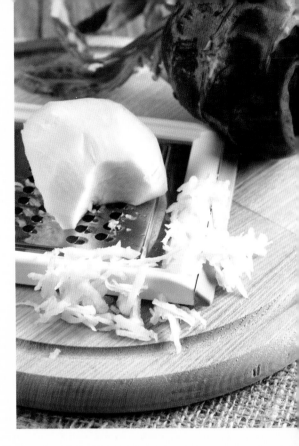

THE NAME KOHLRABI translates as 'turnip cabbage' and the fat round stems taste like a milder, sweeter cross between the two.

Young kohlrabi is delicious eaten raw, sliced into salads, or served alongside other crudites with a dip or vinaigrette. It can also be steamed or roasted, which deepens the flavour. Nothing need go to waste as the leaves are edible too, and can be used in the same way as spinach, chard or kale.

For a fantastic side dish, try this Asian-inspired coleslaw, which makes a lively, healthy change from the usual mayonnaise-drenched concoctions. Great with barbecues, or even as a main served with rice.

Zingy (kohl) slaw
- **1 kohlrabi, coarsely grated**
- **3 carrots, coarsely grated**
- **1 red onion, thinly sliced**
- **1 red pepper, thinly sliced**
- **1 handful of coriander, torn**
- **1 red chilli, finely chopped** (optional)
- **2 tablespoons roasted peanuts, chopped, to finish**

Dressing
- **2 tablespoons sesame oil**
- **2 tablespoons olive oil**
- **2 tablespoons soy sauce** (or fish sauce if you prefer)
- **2 tablespoons lime juice** (or lemon juice)
- **1 garlic clove, finely chopped**
- **1 tablespoon brown sugar**
- **2 tablespoons white wine vinegar or rice vinegar**

Method
• Grate and chop all the veg and throw it into a bowl.

• Whisk together all the dressing ingredients and pour over the veg. Give it all a good stir and top with the roasted peanuts.

Leeks

♥ Love them

Smooth, sleek leeks are a mild-tasting member of the allium family and share the same health-promoting properties as onions and garlic. These hardy vegetables are a natural diuretic and are full of vitamins and minerals. They can be thrown into all sorts of recipes: soups, casseroles, pasta dishes and all things cheesy – with the possible exception of cheesecake.

Leeks have been cultivated for thousands of years and have traditionally been used to relieve many conditions – from the common cold to the pain of childbirth. They were even thought to deter evil spirits.

These days, leeks are valued for their culinary uses and health properties. They are rich in vitamins A and K, and are a good source of vitamins C and B6, iron, folate, magnesium and calcium. And while the thick white stems are prized by chefs, the green parts are also highly nutritious and delicious.

In addition, leeks are rich in a plant chemical called kaempferol. This is a flavanoid which is known to have anti-inflammatory properties and many studies have suggested kaempferol may play a role in combating cancer.[38] Kaempferol is also thought to help relax blood vessels and has been linked to a reduced risk of many conditions, including neurodegenerative diseases like Alzheimer's and Parkinson's, as well as heart disease.[39,40]

And along with garlic and onions, leeks contain the sulphur compound, allicin. This too, is the subject of much research due to its exciting potential in the field of cancer treatment.[41]

They are rich in vitamins A and K, and are a good source of vitamins C and B6, iron, folate, magnesium and calcium ...

❈ Grow them

Leeks are one of those amazing vegetables that will shrug off whatever winter throws at them, to provide valuable food when you need it most. And the less you have to rely on out-of-season, hot-house imports the better.

Growing your own leeks is easy, as long as you follow two basic rules – plant them twice and make the holes really big.

Sowing

In March or April, sow the seeds outdoors in a narrow drill, in a finely raked seedbed. Don't worry too much about location, as you will need to dig them up and move them a few weeks later, anyway. If you want to get a head start you could start the seeds off in containers indoors in January or February, but I find it easier to wait until spring.

Planting

In June, or once the seedlings are 10-15cm tall and look like wispy spring onions, it's time to transplant them to their final home. Dig them up and tease them apart. Some people like to trim the roots and the tops of the leaves, but there's debate about whether this is really necessary. (You can also buy pre-grown seedlings if you didn't get round to sowing your own.)

To transplant leeks, you need to 'dib them in'. This sounds like something a boy scout might do, but simply involves poking a big hole in the earth. There are special tools designed for this very task called 'dibbers', but a fat stick or the handle of a garden tool will do just as well, so don't splash out if you don't have one.

Before creating your holes, water the soil generously, then push the stick (or dibber) into the ground. Wiggle it around until you have a decent hole; about 15cm deep and 5cm wide. Leave 15cm between each hole.

Drop a seedling into each hole and fill with water. Keep doing this until you have used up all your seedlings – or run out of space, whichever happens first.

Don't be tempted to refill the holes with soil. The seedlings should be rattling around like pencils in an empty pot, so they have space to fatten out, otherwise you will end up with a row of skinny waifs.

As the leeks grow, pile some earth around the stems to block out the light. This keeps them white. But if appearances don't worry you, don't bother.

Harvest your leeks through the winter as and when you need them, they will store much better in soil than in the fridge.

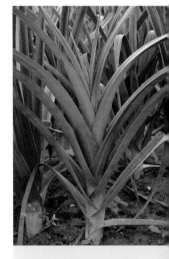

Varieties to try:

'Musselburgh' – a popular, reliable variety.

'The Lyon' – known for its long stems.

'Bleu de Solaise' – a French heritage variety with distinctive bluey-purple leaves. Extremely hardy.

'Apollo' – vigorous, uniform plants with good tolerance to rust.

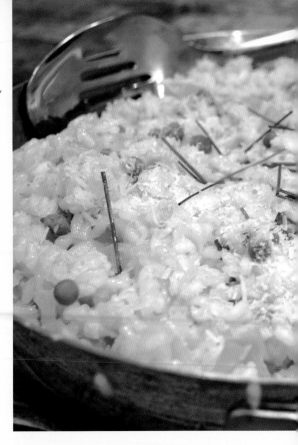 Eat them

LEEK AND POTATO soup is my standby winter supper. It's so easy it's hardly worth including the recipe: just fry leeks and celery, then add some potatoes. Pour in some stock and simmer until the potatoes are soft, before blending. For something slightly more indulgent, this creamy risotto is like a hug on a plate.

Leek and pea risotto

Serves 4

- **4 medium leeks, washed and thinly sliced**
- **30g butter, plus a little extra to finish**
- **1 tablespoon olive oil**
- **300g Arborio risotto rice**
- **200g peas**
- **150ml white wine**
- **Approx 1 litre chicken or vegetable stock**
- **30g Parmesan, grated**
- **2 tablespoons chives, chopped**

Method

- In a saucepan, heat the stock until it's just simmering.

- In a separate pan, melt the butter and oil, then gently sweat the leeks for about 10 minutes until soft and silky.

- Add the rice to the leeks and stir until shiny.

- Turn the heat up a bit. Pour in the wine and stir until it has disappeared.

- Add the stock one ladleful at a time, stirring between each addition so the liquid is absorbed before more is added.

- Keep going until the rice is cooked but slightly al dente – about 20 minutes.

- Boil the peas quickly in a separate pan, then drain and swirl into the risotto.

- Add another knob of butter and stir.

- Season with salt and pepper if necessary, then sprinkle the Parmesan and chives over the top.

- Serve immediately.

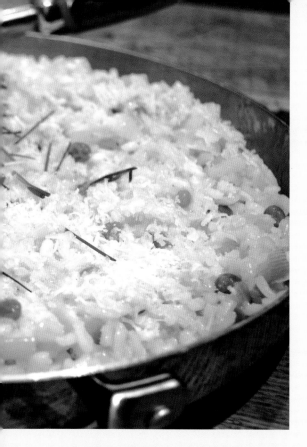

Serves 4
- 3 chunky leeks, sliced
- 4 cloves of garlic, chopped
- 225g cooking chorizo, sliced
- 400g tin butter beans, drained and rinsed
- 100g red lentils
- 2 tablespoons tomato puree
- 500g passata
- 500ml chicken or vegetable stock
- Large handful of kale, torn into fairly small pieces, stalks removed
- Few springs of rosemary

Leek, chorizo and butter bean stew

This hearty, wintery stew is bursting with flavour and nutrients. For a vegetarian version, leave out the chorizo and fry the leeks in olive oil instead.

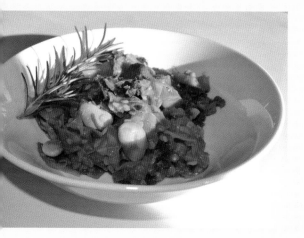

Method

- Dry fry the chorizo on a medium-low heat for a few minutes until the oil is released.

- Add the garlic and leeks and sauté in the chorizo oil for a few minutes, until softened. (Add a splash of olive oil if necessary.)

- Add the lentils, stock, rosemary, passata, butter beans and tomato puree and simmer gently for 20 minutes, or until the lentils are just cooked.

- Add the kale and simmer for another 5 minutes, or until the kale is cooked.

- Turn up the heat and cook on high for a few minutes if you need to reduce the liquid.

- Serve on its own or with crusty bread.

Onions

♥ Love them

Tear-jerkers they may be, but onions are probably the most useful vegetable on the planet. And while they rarely get to star in any dish, they play a supporting role in a multitude of recipes – which is good news considering they come with a stack of nutritional perks. This eye-watering staple has been linked to a range of health benefits from fighting cancer to protecting against diabetes and heart disease.

Like garlic and leeks, onions belong to the allium family and share the same anti-bacterial, anti-fungal and diuretic properties. They are also rich in sulphur compounds and flavonoids. Red onions in particular are a good source of flavonols like quercetin, a powerful antioxidant that has been shown to have anti-cancer and anti-inflammatory properties. Research has indicated that quercetin reduces blood pressure in people with hypertension[42] and studies with animals have shown that it can lower blood sugars.[43]

In addition, onions are high in fibre, and are a source of minerals and vitamins and including vitamins C and B6.

❀ Grow them

For a low-maintenance crop, look no further than onions. Although it is possible to grow them from seed, onions are normally grown from 'sets'. These are small, grape-sized bulbs, that develop into full sized onions.

Onions will survive in most soils, though like all crops they will benefit from some compost or well-rotted manure. This needs to be added in the autumn, rather than at the time of planting, so the bulbs don't rot.

Plant sets outside in March, or early spring. Leave gaps of 8cm between each bulb and 30cm between additional rows. Simply push the bulbs into the soil, fat end first, until the tip is just

This eye-watering staple has been linked to a range of health benefits from fighting cancer to protecting against diabetes and heart disease ...

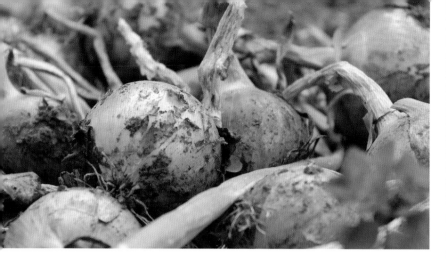

protruding above the soil. Then press the soil down to stop the birds from pulling them out.

Water now and then, but don't overdo it, and try to keep weeds at bay as onions don't like competition.

When the leaves turn yellow and droopy in summer, this is a sign the onions are ready for harvest.

Once you have dug them up, leave them in the sun to dry for a couple of weeks, or bring them indoors if it's likely to rain.

Shallots

Onions are so cheap and readily available, that it may be more worthwhile to grow shallots instead. Closely related to onions, they have a sweeter, more pungent flavour and are more expensive to buy in shops. Plant them in the same way as onions, only a bit earlier in the year, and with slightly larger gaps between them, as they will produce clusters, rather than a single bulb.

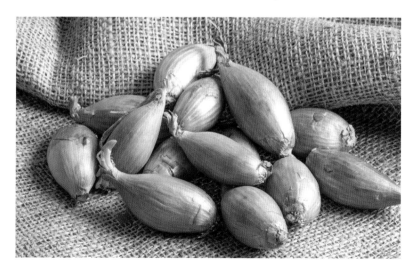

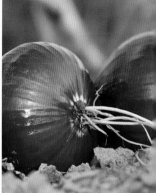

Varieties to try:

'Setton' – a well-known, reliable variety with smooth brown skins.

'Hercules' – produces large onions with dark golden skins.

'Red Baron' – an attractive red variety with a strong flavour and shiny, dark skin.

'Longor' – a shallot with long bulbs and pink-tinted flesh.

Top Tips

☀ Plant onions next to carrots – the allium scent helps to deter the dreaded carrot fly.

☀ If birds are a problem, you may need to cover onions with some kind of netting, especially in the early stages.

✦Eat them

IT'S ALMOST HARDER to avoid
onions, than it is to include them.
They feature in countless casseroles,
curries, stir fries, soups, salads and
more. In most recipes, they merge
unobtrusively into the background.
Yet this incredible onion soup proves
that doesn't have to be the case.

Rich onion soup

Serves 6
- **50g unsalted butter**
- **1 tablespoon olive oil**
- **1kg onions, thinly sliced**
  (red, white or both)
- **4 cloves of garlic, sliced**
- **A few sprigs of fresh thyme**
- **1.2 litres beef stock**
- **275ml red wine**
- **2 bay leaves**
- **Salt and pepper to season**

To serve (optional)
- **Sliced French bread**
- **130g Gruyère cheese, grated**

Method

• Melt the butter and oil in a heavy-
based pan. Add the onions and sauté
slowly over a medium-low heat to
caramelise, for 40 minutes, stirring
frequently.

• Add the garlic, bay and thyme, and
season with a little salt and pepper.
Cook gently for another 15 minutes.

• Turn up the heat, add the wine and
boil until the liquid has evaporated.

• Pour in the stock and simmer for
40 minutes. Season to taste.

• Toast the bread under a grill, then
melt the cheese on top. Serve with
the soup.

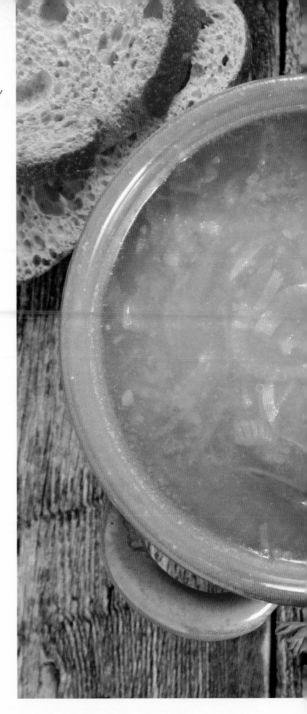

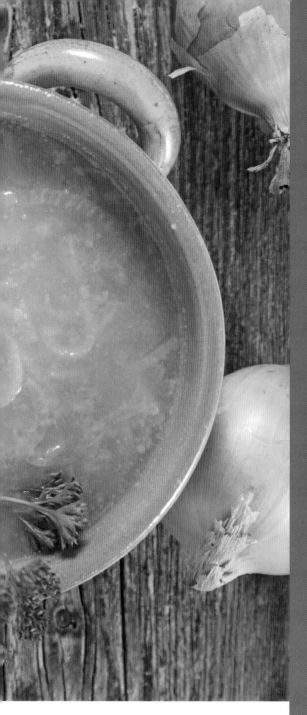

Onion bhajis

Makes 10-12
- 100g gram (chickpea) flour
- 1 large onion, finely shredded
- ½ teaspoon cumin
- ½ teaspoon garam masala
- ½ teaspoon ground turmeric
- ¼ teaspoon salt
- Water
- Vegetable oil

Method

- Combine the flour and spices in a bowl. Add enough water to make a sticky batter.

- Mix in the shredded onion.

- Pour the oil into a heavy-based pan, so that it's about 1cm deep.

- Take spoonfuls of the batter, flatten slightly, then fry for about two minutes on each side until crisp and golden.

- Place on kitchen paper to absorb the excess oil and serve with mango chutney or natural yoghurt.

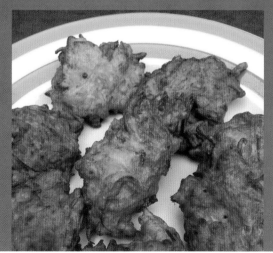

Peas

♥ Love them

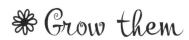

Fresh and frozen peas are so incomparable they could almost be two different vegetables. As soon as peas are picked the sugars start changing to starches, so freshness is measured in minutes rather than days, hence the reliance on frozen varieties. Even the fresh peas sold in shops are nothing like the ones you can pick yourself. The only way to discover the true taste of peas is to grow your own and it's practically obligatory to eat some of them straight from the pod. No cooking required.

Besides being a crop that money can't buy, peas are also extremely good for you. For a start, they are one of the best sources of vegetable protein, making them a valuable ingredient in a vegan or vegetarian diet. The protein also makes them more filling than other vegetables. In addition, peas are loaded with vitamins A, C and K, as well as some B vitamins, especially thiamin (B1) which helps release energy from food, and is important for the nervous and digestive systems.

Peas also contain a useful supply of vitamin B9, or folate. This is needed for the production of red blood cells, and for the healthy development of babies in the womb. What's more, scientists have discovered that people with people with low levels of folate are more likely to suffer from depression[44] so eating peas – along with other natural sources of folate including asparagus, avocados and leafy greens – could benefit your mind as well as your body.

Peas and other leguminous vegetables are also a good source of plant sterols which have been shown to lower LDL (bad) cholesterol, high levels of which are associated with coronary heart disease.[45]

They are one of the best sources of vegetable protein, making them a valuable ingredient in a vegan or vegetarian diet ...

❀ Grow them

Peas are extremely pleasing to grow, and an ideal crop to grow with children. The large seeds are easy for small hands to handle, and there is nothing quite like picking and popping the pods a few months later. Just don't expect them to leave any for you.

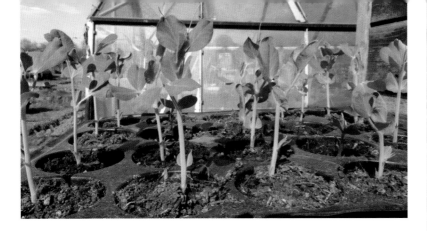

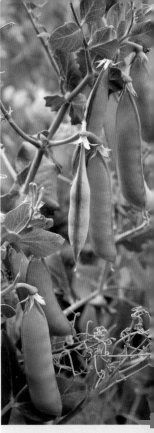

Sowing

Peas are usually sown from March. You can start them off indoors in pots, or toilet rolls, and transplant them outdoors when they are around 10cm high.

Another technique is to sow peas in a piece of guttering filled with potting compost, then slide the contents into the ground once the seedlings are established.

But if it's not too cold or wet, peas can also be planted directly into the ground and this is the easiest option of all. Pick a warm, dry day, then make a narrow trench, about 3cm deep and 20cm wide. Water it, then press the seeds in at 5cm intervals, cover them over with soil, and wait for them to grow.

Aftercare

As the seedlings grow, they produce wispy tendrils which look for something to twirl around, so you will need to have some supports in place. Rustic twigs are the most attractive option, but if you don't have any at your disposal, netting or chicken wire also works. Plant a row of peas on either side, so you get two rows for the price of one.

The peas should be ready to harvest within three months, once the pods are nice and plump. You can also eat the shoots which are delicious in salads.

At the end of the season, cut the plants down to just above ground level, but leave the roots underground as these add valuable nitrogen to the soil.

Problems and how to avoid them

Birds, slugs and mice are all partial to pea seeds, so sow generously as an insurance policy – you can always thin them out if they all survive. If incumbent wildlife are a particular pest, try covering the seeds with upturned jam jars, plastic bottles cut in half, or chicken wire placed over the ground.

Varieties to try:

'Kelvedon Wonder' – a very popular variety and a prolific cropper that only grows about one metre tall.

'Feltham First' – a traditional variety that produces lots of long pods with sweet-tasting peas.

'Waverex' – a petit pois type that produces tiny, sweet-tasting peas.

'Oregon Sugar Pod' – a delicious mangetout variety.

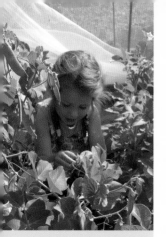

Top Tips

☀ Sow a new row of seeds every four weeks until July, to provide a continuous harvest.

☀ Snip off the top growing shoots of each plant when they are about 30cm high to encourage more pods to develop.

☀ As well as regular peas, it's worth trying a few sugar snaps and mangetout, which can be grown in the same way. Look out for unusual varieties, such as purple ones, to spice up your plot.

☀ For an early harvest, peas can be sown in autumn and kept undercover until spring. This is a bit more ambitious, but choosing the right variety will give the best chance of success.

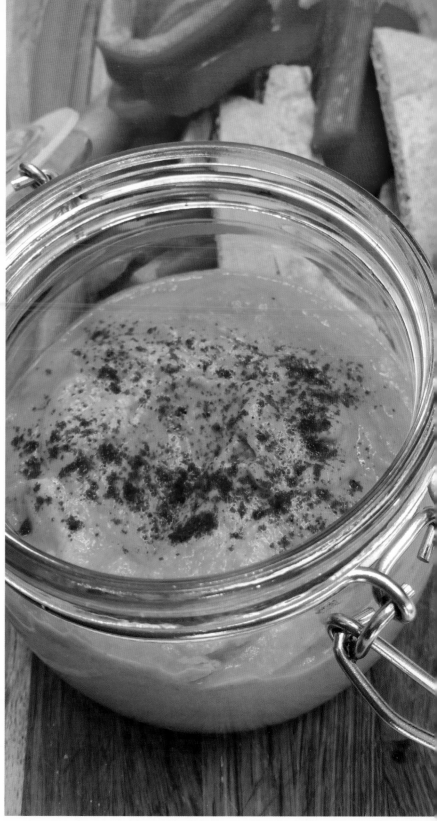

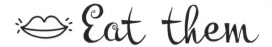 # Eat them

PART OF THE joy of growing peas is eating them straight from the pods, like little green sweets. If you still have some left after that, they are brilliant scattered in salads, either raw or barely boiled.

Green hummus

Is it a dip, is it a spread, is it hummus? The jury's out but it's a yes for taste.

- **400g peas**
- **3 cloves of garlic, crushed**
- **1 tablespoon tahini**
- **Juice of one lemon**
- **Pinch of salt**
- **Handful of walnuts, chopped into small pieces**
- **A sprinkling of smoked paprika**

Method

• Cook the peas in boiling, salted water for two minutes. Refresh under cold water.

• Whizz the peas, garlic, tahini, lemon juice and salt in a blender. Add a drop of olive oil if it's a bit on the dry side. Stir in the walnuts and sprinkle with smoked paprika.

• Serve as a dip with veg sticks and pita strips, or smother onto oatcakes.

Simple pea, bean and puy lentil salad with honey and mustard dressing

Serves 4–6
- **250g peas**
- **250g french beans**
- **185g puy lentils**
- **750ml vegetable stock** (or water)

For the dressing
- **3 tablespoons lemon juice**
- **2 teaspoons honey**
- **2 teaspoons dijon mustard**
- **6 tablespoons olive oil**
- **1 clove garlic, crushed**
- **Salt and pepper**

Method

• Rinse and drain the lentils, then place in the saucepan with the stock (or water.) Bring to the boil and simmer for 20-25 minutes. They should still have some bite to them. Drain and place in a bowl.

• Blanch the peas and beans in boiling water until just tender. Drain and refresh under cold water.

• Toss the peas and beans with the lentils.

• For the dressing, whisk all the ingredients together, or shake in a jam jar with the lid firmly closed, then pour over the salad.

Raspberries

❤ Love them

Although sometimes a second favourite to strawberries, raspberries contain a mega-mix of nutrients and antioxidants. These health-enhancing berries could help slow down the ageing process, reduce the risk of many diseases and even protect your joints.

What's more, raspberries are naturally low in sugar and are one of the top scoring fruits and vegetables when it comes to fibre. This is because one raspberry is composed of lots of individual fruits, or drupelets, all clustered together, each with its own seed. Raspberries are also packed with vitamin C and are a good source of copper, manganese, potassium, folate and vitamins K and E.

Like other berries, they contain a super supply of antioxidants. Two of the most beneficial substances found in raspberries are ellagic acid and anthocyanins – the pigments responsible for the red colour. Lots of research has been carried out into the potential benefits of these and other important compounds, and evidence suggests they could help to protect against many chronic conditions, especially cardiovascular disease, diabetes, obesity, Alzheimers and cancer.[46]

Raspberries could also offer a natural remedy for rheumatoid arthritis, as they are known to have anti-inflammatory effects. It's still early days as far as research is concerned, but there is hope that regularly eating raspberries could be beneficial for joint health.

There is also a considerable buzz around the black raspberry, a blackberry-raspberry combo which is which is said to have exceptionally high levels of ellagic acid, anthocyanins and antioxidants. There is much excitement about the potential anti-cancer properties of this unusual fruit and various trials have shown that black raspberry extract can inhibit the growth of tumours.[47] You might not be able to buy black raspberries in shops, but the canes are available online and this could be a variety that's well worth including for both health and flavour.

Raspberries could also offer a natural remedy for rheumatoid arthritis, as they are known to have anti-inflammatory effects ...

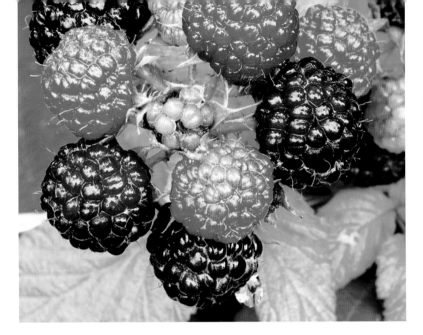

Black raspberries. have exceptionally high levels of ellagic acid, anthocyanins and antioxidants.

❋ Grow them

There are two main types of raspberries: summer fruiting and autumn fruiting. Both are simple to grow and require little maintenance. The autumn ones are the easiest of all and seem to be less of a target for birds. But if you have space to grow both types, you will have fresh raspberries at your fingertips for even longer.

Raspberry canes are a great investment as they will carry on producing fruit for around 10 years, which is even better when you consider the cost of shop-bought punnets. And of course, growing your own means you can try varieties that money can't buy, including the supercharged black ones, and luxurious looking gold ones.

Planting

Raspberries grow well in cool, damp climates and will do best in fertile, well-drained soil.

Both summer and autumn raspberries grow on canes. These can be planted from autumn to early spring, as long as the ground isn't waterlogged or frozen.

Ideally, dig some well-rotted manure or garden compost into the soil before planting. Soak the roots in water, then make large holes in the ground. Sink the canes into the holes so the roots are below ground level, leaving about 45 cm between each cane. If they look

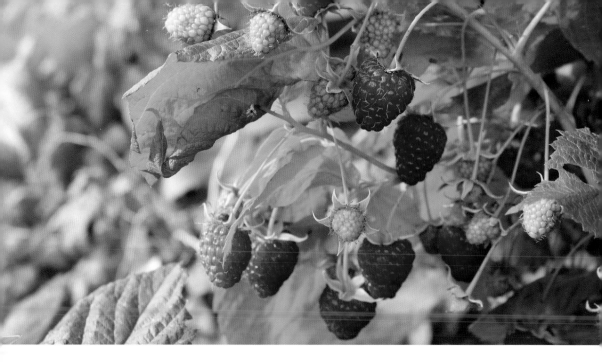

a bit lanky, trim them down so they are about 20cm high.

In spring, spread some compost or manure around the canes and water during dry spells.

Summer-fruiting raspberries

These produce fruit on canes that grew the previous year, so are already one year old. This means you won't get any raspberries during the first summer, but it's worth that frustrating wait. The following year, and every year after that, your canes should be dripping with raspberries. Enjoy!

In autumn, remove all the canes that bore fruit by cutting them down to soil level. Leave the rest of the canes (the new, green ones) alone as these will produce fruit the following year.

Summer varieties of raspberries need some support to help them stand up. A good system is to hammer a few wooden posts into the ground, then stretch three rows of parallel wires between the posts. As the fruit canes grow, tie them to the wires to stop them from sprawling over the ground.

Autumn-fruiting raspberries

Autumn varieties produce fruit on new wood every year, and can be harvested from August to October just as most other soft fruit is coming to an end, so they are a great crop for extending the berry season.

In winter, chop all the canes right back to the ground. This seems

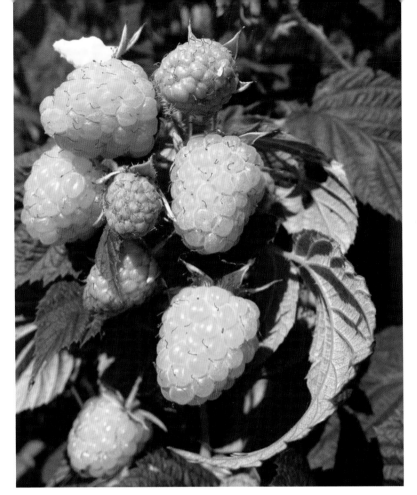

Autumn Gold
raspberries.

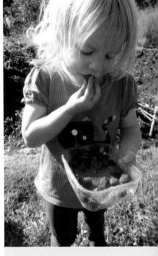

ruthless, but new shoots will emerge the following spring and produce more fruit. Autumn varieties produce shorter, sturdier canes so they shouldn't need any support.

Both summer and autumn raspberries produce suckers, or new shoots, that appear in random locations around existing plants. You can leave these where they are as long as it's not too crowded, or dig them up and replant them in a more orderly fashion. If you don't have room for any more, cut them down or dig them up and give them away to friends.

Problems

Summer raspberries are often a target for birds, so cover plants with netting if necessary. An easy way to do this is to attach a piece of wood to the top of the support posts to make a 'T' shape, then throw the netting over the top. There's no need to splash out on anything expensive – old net curtains from charity shops will do the job just as well, despite looking a little flouncy.

Varieties to try:

Summer varieties to try:
'Glen Ample' – one of the heaviest cropping midsummer varieties, with flavoursome berries and spine-free canes.

'Tulameen' – produces deliciously sweet, large fruit in midsummer.

Autumn varieties to try:
'Autumn Bliss' – a heavy cropping, popular variety.

'Autumn Gold' – produces delicious gold-coloured fruits. Guaranteed to impress.

⋙ Eat them

LIKE MOST SUMMER fruits, raspberries don't really need embellishing. There's little you can do to improve on that just-picked aromatic sweetness, especially if you want to keep it healthy. However, summer days call for ice-cream, so it's always good to have some stashed in the freezer. If you've never tried making ice-cream using condensed milk before, prepare to be amazed. This is a doddle to whip up and so creamy, and you don't need an ice-cream maker. Just don't reveal your secret ingredient.

No churn raspberry ice-cream

- **400g fresh raspberries**
- **A squeeze of lemon juice**
- **405g tin condensed milk**
- **300ml whipping cream**

Method

Whizz the raspberries in a blender to make a puree. Add a squeeze of lemon juice to bring out the flavour. Press the puree through a sieve if you want to go seedless.

- Whisk the cream and condensed milk together until you get soft peaks.

- Swirl the raspberry puree through the creamy mixture.

- Transfer to a freezable container and freeze for a few hours or overnight.

Raspberry and yoghurt ice lollies

For a lighter alternative to ice-cream these ice-lollies double up as a refreshing dessert or a healthy snack. Definitely not just for children. And of course, you can use other fruit besides raspberries.

Makes 8
- **50g caster sugar**
- **250g raspberries**
- **500ml Greek-style yoghurt**
- **1 teaspoon vanilla paste** (or extract)

Method

- Place the raspberries and sugar in a bowl. Cover and leave to stand for half an hour or so, then mash with a fork. Stir in the vanilla.

- Swirl the raspberries through the yogurt, then pour into lolly moulds and place in the freezer until solid.

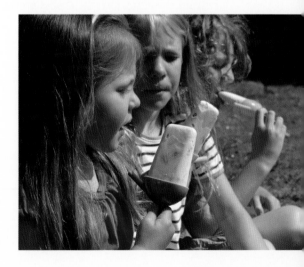

Salad

♥ Love it

The terms salad and lettuce are used synonymously to encompass a multitude of edible leaves as the insipid iceberg is eclipsed by an ever-expanding range of bagged leaves. This may seem like a step forward for flavour and diversity, but it's really just a token gesture. For the price of a bag of ready-to-eat garnish (there's never enough for much more than that) you could buy a packet of seeds and have your own continuous supply of super fresh, super nutritious leaves throughout the year, packaged in nothing more than soil and fresh air. And you will be avoiding all those pesticides in the process.

Salad leaves are one of the easiest crops to grow yourself, and you get stacks of return for your money. You don't even need a garden, they will do just as well, if not better, in containers. Five minutes and a windowsill is all it takes.

Generally speaking, the greener the salad, the higher the level of nutrients, with bonus points if there's a bit of red in there too. So forget icebergs and opt for varieties like Lollo Rossa and Romaine. These and other strongly coloured varieties are a great source of vitamins K and A, as well as some vitamin C, folate and other minerals. Growing as many different varieties as you can will ensure you get a range of nutrients. Try Asian greens like Bok Choy and Pak Choi which are rich in iron and calcium, rocket which is packed with antioxidants, and more unusual flavours like chicory and endives. For a real super salad, it has to be home grown.

Salad leaves are one of the easiest crops to grow yourself, and you get stacks of return for your money ...

❋ Grow it

There are two main kinds of salad crops; the familiar lettuces with a central heart that you pick once like Romaine and Butterheads, and loose-leaf types like lamb's lettuce, mizuna and rocket, which are also known as and cut-and-come-again varieties and provide a continuous supply of leaves. With a little planning, you can eat home-grown salad all year round, it's just a case of knowing what to sow and when.

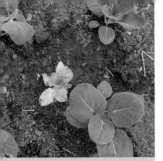

Intercropping lettuces between other plants makes good use of space.

Top Tips

☼ Sow a handful of seeds every few weeks for a continuous supply of leaves.

☼ Sow lettuces in between other, bigger crops to make good use of space. The larger crops will also provide useful shade during the summer.

☼ Harvest leaves in early morning or during the evening, to get them at their freshest.

☼ For summer sowings, sow seeds in the evening when it's cooler, as they won't germinate in hot temperatures.

☼ Don't let the soil dry out, as this increases the risk of bolting.

☼ Cover winter varieties with a cloche or fleece for added protection.

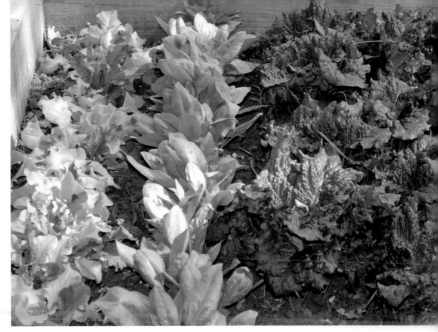

Salad grows well in raised beds.

Start a few seeds off indoors in February and plant out from March. Then sow batches of seed outdoors every few weeks during spring and summer. In autumn, sow hardy (cold tolerant) varieties like 'Winter Density' and 'Marvel of Four Seasons' that will survive the winter to provide crops the following spring.

How to plant

Salad crops will grow well even in poor quality soil, but if you can add some garden compost or manure before sowing they will do even better.

For quick and simple results, try a cut-and-come-again variety. These types are ideal for growing in containers and can be ready to eat in a matter of weeks. Container grown salads are extremely easy to manage and are often less of a target for slugs.

There are hundreds of different types of salad leaves and lettuces to choose from. Check the packet for sowing times and instructions, as this will vary depending on the variety. Most varieties can be sown anytime between spring and summer. But you can also sow some types in the autumn which will help to extend the picking season.

Sprinkle the seeds thinly onto damp soil or compost and cover over lightly. Don't allow the ground to dry out.

For traditional hearting types of lettuce, it can help to sow the seeds in pots or trays first and plant them out once the seedlings are big enough to handle. This gives you a bit more control as it's easy to get overrun by hundreds of tiny seedlings. Alternatively, just sow seed directly into the ground and thin the seedlings out to leave others to grow to full size. The thinnings can also be eaten, of course.

Problems

The number one enemy of lettuce is the loathsome slug. These slimy molluscs can end your salad days in one brutal night, blithely munching through an entire row of seedlings. This is another good reason to grow at least some of your salad crops in containers. They won't be completely immune, but they will be less vulnerable.

There are all sorts of tactics you can employ in slug warfare, including: beer traps, copper tape, crushed egg shells and coffee grinds. Or try tempting some toads and hedgehogs into your garden for a midnight feast. Failing that, there is some grisly satisfaction to be derived from snipping slugs in half with a sharp pair of scissors – although you may need to stay up all night to make a significant dent in the population.

If the above measures don't work (and there's a good chance they won't) then nematodes may well be the answer. These are microscopic organisms that can be applied to the soil using a watering can for an effective, organic way of controlling slugs.

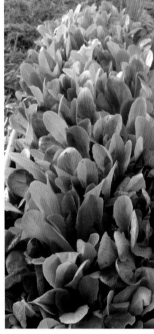

Salad grown in containers is less vulnerable to slugs.

Varieties to try:

Salad Bowl – a popular and productive loose-leaf variety with red or green leaves.

Lollo Rossa – an easy to grow loose-leaf Italian variety with frilly green and red leaves for spring and summer sowings.

Rocket – the famously peppery leaves are one of the first salad crops to mature in spring. Sow in early spring and then every few weeks until late summer and harvest until early winter.

Oriental mixes – look out for mixed packets of seeds containing different varieties like Mizuna, Mibuna, Mustard Greens and Tatsoi. Can be grown most of the year.

Varieties for picking during winter:

'Artic King' – a large, extremely hardy Butterhead type of lettuce.

Winter Purslane – hardy and tasty leaves that can be sown in August and September and picked throughout the winter.

Land Cress – similar to watercress and can be picked throughout winter. Cover it with fleece if it gets really cold.

Lamb's Lettuce – also known as corn salad. Mild tasting leaves that will keep going through the winter.

'Winter Density' – a hardy variety of lettuce with crisp leaves. Seeds can be sown in autumn for a spring harvest.

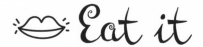 # Eat it

HAVING A HARVEST-READY supply of salad at your disposal is one of the easiest ways to bump up your daily quota of fruit and veg without even trying. A handful of leaves on the side of the plate is like a side-helping of vitamins for no extra effort. But for a real health-kick, don't make an accessory out of salad, let it take over the plate instead.

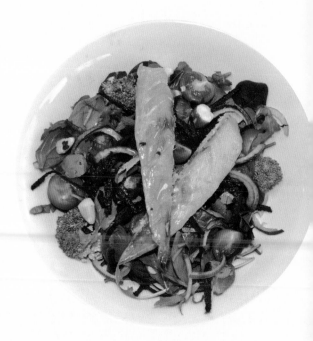

Feel good salad

This mood-boosting salad is packed with nutrients that are great for both mind and body, including lots of B vitamins from the fish and greens. A deficiency of B vitamins – especially B12 (found mainly in animal products) B6 and B9 (folate) – has been linked to depression.[44] The mackerel provides brain-boosting omega-3 fats along with with vitamin D, which is rarely found in foods, and both of these substances can also affect mood. The brazil nuts provide selenium which is important for many bodily processes, inlcuding thyroid function, and selenium may also support mental health.

Serves 4
- **250g mixed salad leaves or a head of lettuce**
- **Handful of spinach leaves**
- **Handful of tomatoes, halved or chopped**
- **2 raw beetroot, peeled**
- **250g broccoli**
- **½ red onion, finely sliced**
- **4 smoked mackerel fillets**
- **Large handful of brazil nuts, roughly chopped**
- **Splash of olive oil**
- **Squeeze of lemon juice**

Method

• Steam the broccoli for 3 or 4 minutes until just tender. Grate the beetroot.

• Combine the salad leaves, tomatoes, onion, broccoli and spinach in a large bowl.

• Top with the brazil nuts and beetroot, but don't mix, and serve with the mackerel on top.

• Drizzle with olive oil and a squeeze of lemon juice.

Spinach

♥ Love it

Vegetables don't come much greener than spinach, and anything with that much chlorophyll has to be good for you. No wonder Popeye loved it – despite the unappetizing appeal of the tinned variety. Fortunately, fresh spinach has a lot more going for it – both in terms of taste and nutrition.

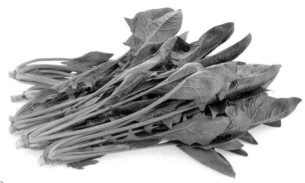

It might not give you cartoon biceps, but it is packed with vitamins, minerals and antioxidants, for a powerful health kick.

Spinach provides vast amounts of vitamin A (from carotenoids) which is needed for healthy skin and eyes. It's also a great source of vitamins C, K and E, and loads of minerals. Gram for gram, the dark green leaves contain around twice as much potassium as bananas. You will also get magnesium, manganese, zinc, calcium and of course iron – although perhaps not quite as much as we have been led to believe. 100 grams of spinach contains 1.89g of iron, compared to 2.3g in 100 grams of fillet steak.[16] Plant-derived iron is harder for the body to absorb than iron found in meat, but take-up is improved if it's consumed along with some vitamin C – of which spinach itself is a source.

In addition, spinach contains super concentrations of disease-fighting antioxidants, including alpha-lipoic acid (ALA) which is thought to help protect the body against many chronic conditions from cancer to diabetes.[48] Spinach also provides the antioxidants lutein and zeathanthin, which are essential for eye health and preventing cataracts.

The list of potential health benefits of spinach is almost endless, making it a prudent choice for any veg patch or allotment. It's fair to say the pipe-smoking sailor man knew what was good for him – apart from nicotine, that is.

Gram for gram, the dark green leaves contain around twice as much potassium as bananas ...

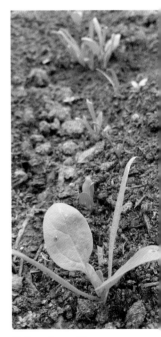

Spinach seedlings.

❋ Grow it

Spinach is easy and quick to grow and will happily put up with shade and cool conditions, but in hot weather it can bolt, or turn

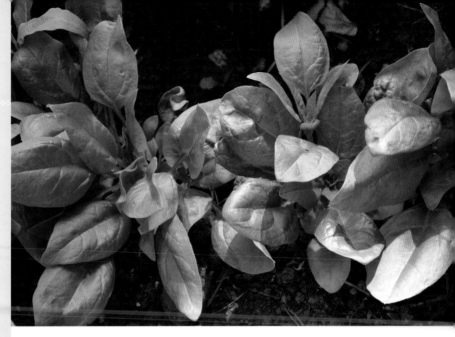

Varieties to try:

'Emilia' – fast-growing and tasty with good disease resistance.

'Matador' – slow to bolt so good for summer sowings.

'Reddy' – a fast-growing versatile variety with attractive red stems.

'Giant Winter' – a very hardy variety, which produces leaves in autumn and winter.

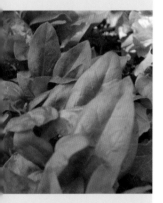

Top Tips

☀ In summer, try sowing spinach seeds in between larger crops like brassicas. As well as making use of empty space, the larger crops will also provide spinach with some shade protection.

to flower, as soon as your back is turned. With a bit of planning you can harvest your own spinach almost all year round. It likes rich, fertile soil, so apply a generous helping of compost or manure before sowing.

Sow seeds every four weeks from March to October, selecting varieties to suit the time of year, and sprinkle them thinly into drills that are about 2cm deep.

Baby leaves can be ready in a matter of weeks, depending on the conditions. Pick them little and often and they will keep growing back. Or you can harvest the whole plant when it's bigger, in which case thin the seedlings out as they grow until there are 15cm gaps between them.

Spinach needs plenty of water especially during hot summers, when it's very prone to bolting, so it's best to pick it as baby leaves during this period. If it does run to flower, the leaves will turn bitter, so just pull them up and start again.

Problems and how to avoid them

Downy mildew – this is a fungal infection that causes leaves to turn blotchy and mouldy. It flourishes in warm, damp conditions, so leave room for air to circulate between plants to reduce the risk, and get rid of any affected leaves as soon as you spot them.

Rabbits seem to have an uncanny knack for sniffing out spinach from about five miles away. And then they will munch on whatever else is on offer too. If necessary, protect plants with netting, electric fences, angry dogs, or whatever it takes.

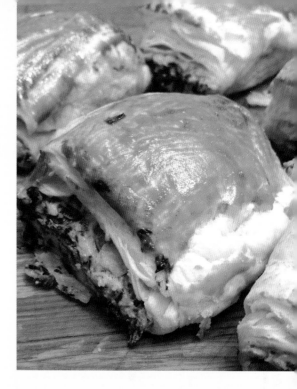

✦ Eat it

FOR MAXIMUM HEALTH benefits, throw copious amounts of raw, bright spinach into salads with a splash of olive oil plus lemon juice to help with the absorption of fat-soluble vitamins and iron. For a party piece or quick lunch, these sausage-less rolls are a hit with vegetarians and meat-eaters alike. I cheat and buy the puff pastry, but of course you could make your own.

Sausage-less rolls

Spinach and ricotta were made to go together. And the puff pastry provides the perfect packaging.

Makes 12-15
- **250g fresh spinach**
- **250g ricotta**
- **500g puff pastry**
- **50g pine nuts**
- **1 clove of garlic, crushed**
- **2 egg yolks**
- **1 whole egg, beaten**
- **50g cheddar cheese**
- **¼ teaspoon grated nutmeg**
- **1 teaspoon lemon zest**
- **Handful of chives, chopped**

Method

- Preheat the oven to 180°C/160°C fan/gas mark 3.

- Heat a small frying pan and dry fry the pine nuts until golden brown. Set them aside.

- Throw the spinach into the pan and cook until just wilted. Add a tiny bit of water if necessary, but no more than a few drops.

- Transfer the spinach to a bowl and allow to cool. Then add the pine nuts, egg yolks, ricotta, cheddar, lemon zest, chives and nutmeg. Stir until well combined and season.

- Roll the pastry out into a large thin rectangle, then cut into two long rectangles.

- Place a mound of filling along the middle of each rectangle, leaving enough space around the edge to bring the sides of the pastry together. Then brush each rectangle with beaten egg on one side.

- Fold the opposite side of the pastry onto the egg-washed side and press down to seal. Do this for both rectangles.

- Slice each pastry roll into about 8 smaller rolls and place on a baking tray, sealed side down. Brush with beaten egg.

- Cook for 40 minutes, or until crisp and golden.

Spinach calzone

The literal meaning of calzone is 'big sock.' It is of course a folded pizza, that resembles a large pasty – or a sock, depending on your point of view. One advantage of folding your pizza is that the filling can't slide off.

Makes 3 calzones
- **300g strong white flour**
- **7g fast-action dried yeast**
- **1 teaspoon of salt**
- **200ml warm water**
- **2 tablespoons olive oil**
- **2 x 150g fresh mozzarella, cut into small cubes**
- **100g fresh spinach, chopped**

Method

• Prepare the dough by combining the flour, yeast and salt in a large bowl. Make a well in the centre and add the warm water and oil. Mix everything together to make a wet dough. Tip onto a work surface and knead for 5-10 minutes until smooth and elastic. Add more flour if it's too wet and sticking to your hands. (You can also make the dough in a machine with a dough hook if you have one.)

• Place the dough in an oiled bowl and cover with clingfilm or a damp tea towel. Leave in a warm place to rise for about an hour, or until the dough has doubled in size.

• Meanwhile dice the mozzarella into small cubes and place in a sieve over a bowl, to allow the liquid to drain off.

• Preheat the oven to 220°C/fan 200°C/gas 6.

• Turn the dough out onto a floured surface and knock out the air by giving it a quick knead.

• Divide the dough into three balls and leave for another 20 minutes.

• When risen again, roll the dough out into circles about 20-25cm in diameter, then place on an oiled baking tray.

• Scatter the diced mozzarella and chopped spinach on one half of each calzone, leaving 1cm around the edge for sealing. Fold the uncovered half of the dough over the filling and press the edges together to make a hem around the outside.

• Place in the oven for around 20 minutes until golden.

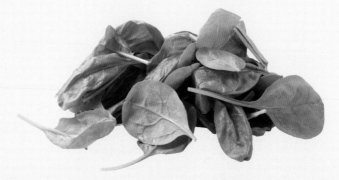

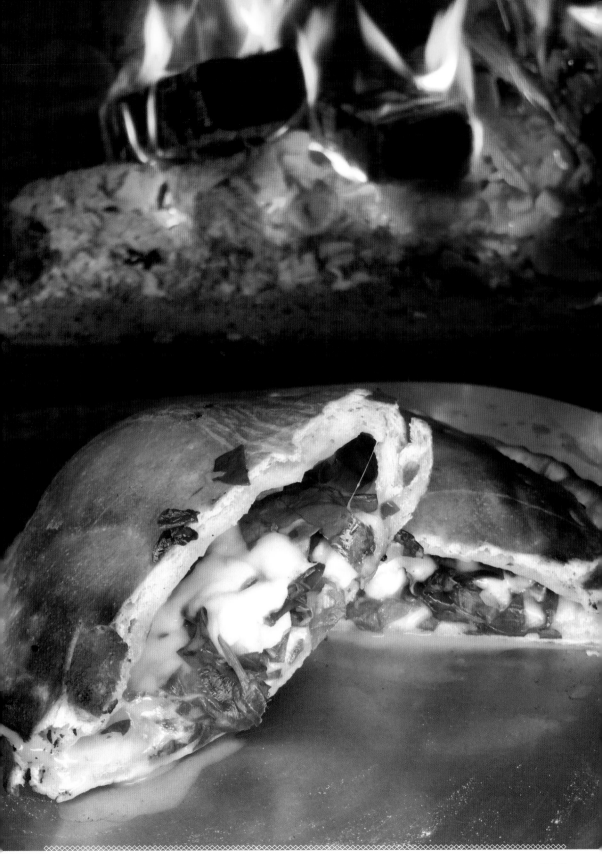

Squashes and pumpkins

♥ Love them

Winter squashes and pumpkins come in all shapes and sizes but share a communal podium of health benefits. Beneath the tough exteriors, the vivid orange flesh is an impressive source of beta-carotene and other carotenoids which are converted into vitamin A in the body. Butternut is the most commonly eaten winter squash, and provides even more vitamin A than other varieties. A single serving will give you more than twice the amount, or RNI, needed per day.

Don't worry about overdosing though. Unlike preformed vitamin A – found in meat, fish and dairy products – excessive amounts of beta-carotene are not thought to be toxic, as the body simply converts less into vitamin A. In extreme cases, beta-carotene can give the skin an orange tinge, although this is harmless and reversible. As well as beta-carotene, squashes and pumpkins also contain some rarer carotenoids, like alpha carotene and beta-cryptoxanthin which are powerful antioxidants.

To top it off, squashes are good source of vitamin C, as well as B vitamins and a number of important minerals including potassium, magnesium and manganese.

And don't forget the seeds. These can be baked to form a high-fibre nutritious snack, rich in heart-happy mono-unsaturated fatty acids, protein, magnesium and zinc which is important for the immune system, fertility, and prostate health in men. And for incurable insomniacs the seeds are good source of tryptophan, a natural sleeping aid.

> As well as beta-carotene, squashes and pumpkins also contain some rarer carotenoids, like alpha carotene and beta-cryptoxanthin which are powerful antioxidants ...

❀ Grow them

For home-grown wow factor, pumpkins and squashes are hard to beat. Children will delight in growing their own monster-sized pumpkins in time for Halloween. However, for culinary purposes, there are tastier, less watery options, so it's worth growing other

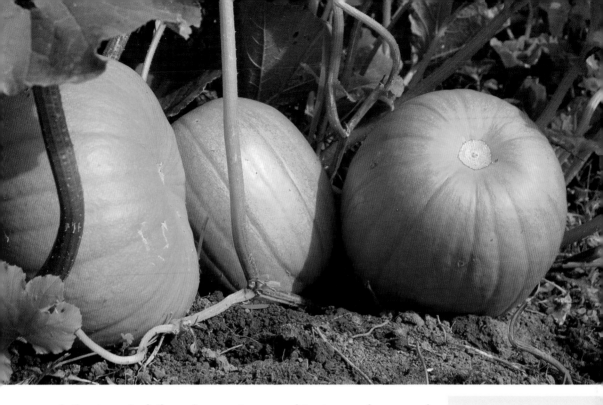

varieties too. And there is a vast array of textures, shapes and colours to choose from, the likes of which are never seen in shops. This is a plant that comes in all sorts of weird and wonderful manifestations; rude, unearthly parodies of the smooth and ordinary butternut known to supermarkets.

Sowing and planting

Despite the variation in appearance, squashes and pumpkins are all grown in the same way and are low-maintenance plants with a good success rate, even for complete beginners. The crucial thing is to start the seeds off indoors, no earlier than April, and don't let the resulting seedlings anywhere near the back door until it's unquestionably T-shirt weather.

Sow seeds 1cm deep in pots of potting compost, by pushing the seed vertically into the soil so it's standing on its edge. This stops it from rotting. Place the pots on a sunny windowsill or inside a propagator, until after germination. If the seedlings become too big, they might need re-potting indoors until it's warm enough to plant them in the ground outside.

In June, assuming the risk of frost has passed, harden the plants off for 7-10 days by taking them outside for a few hours each day. Then plant out in a sunny, sheltered spot and incorporate some manure into the hole. It's a good idea to cover young plants with

Top Tips

☀ As the fruits grow, place them on an old tile or piece of slate to keep them off wet ground.

☀ For a super-sized pumpkin, remove all the fruits except one.

☀ Water generously, especially when the fruits are growing. Like all fruiting vegetables, pumpkins and squashes will benefit from a potassium-rich feed, like comfrey tea.

☀ For even stronger plants, try growing them on an old compost heap.

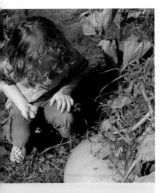

SQUASH

'**Marina di Chioggia**'
– gnarled, green and
warty on the outside;
but silky, sweet and
orange on the inside.

'**Turk's Turban**' – this
bizarre-looking squash
looks like it was grown
in a circus with its
eclectic combination
of stripes, colours and
contours.

Butternut –
predictable, but
delicious none the less.

PUMPKIN

'**Jack O' Lantern**' –
the original carving
model.

'**Honey Bear**' –
produces cute,
miniature pumpkins,
suitable for container
growing.

half a plastic bottle, or the lid of a propagator. This provides added protection against slugs and the elements.

The plants can grow with alarming speed, so leave plenty of space between them (at least a metre) and don't plant them too near other crops or they will suffocate them.

For small gardens, or to free up space on the ground, some varieties of squash can be trained to grow up a frame or trellis. If the fruit becomes too heavy, support it in slings made from netting or old tights, and tied to the frame.

Harvesting

Leave the fruit on the plant for as long as possible, providing there's no chance of frost. When fully grown and the stalk starts to crack, cut the squash or pumpkin free from the plant, with some stem still attached. Place in the sun for about for about 10 days to allow the skin to harden. Most varieties should then store for several months.

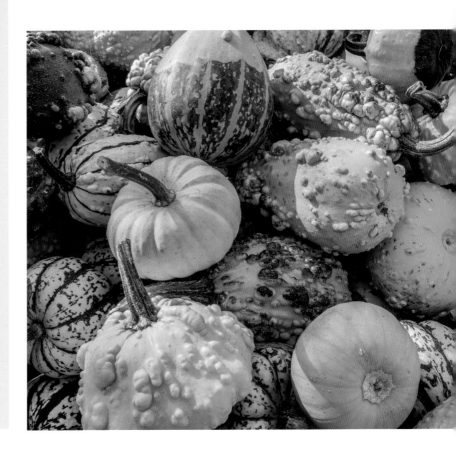

~ Eat them

IN RECENT YEARS, squash has been reinvented as a low-carb apology for pasta. Spiralisers have a lot to answer for. But when left to its own merits, squash shines in stews, soups and risottos, or simply roasted in the oven. It's also surprisingly good in cakes, and makes perfect baby food.

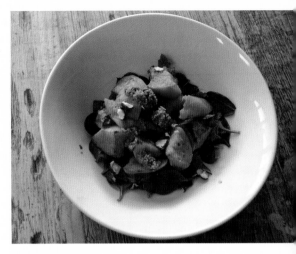

Roast squash with hazelnuts and home-made pesto

- **1 squash**
- **Olive oil**
- **Salt and pepper**
- **2 tablespoons of hazelnuts**

For the pesto
- **60g basil leaves (without stalks)**
- **50g pine nuts**
- **50g Parmesan cheese, grated**
- **1 clove of garlic**
- **Juice of half a lemon**
- **100ml olive oil**
- **Salt to season**

Method

• Preheat the oven to 220°C/fan 200°C/gas 7.

• When the oven is hot, place the hazelnuts on a baking tray and cook for about five minutes until lightly browned. Set aside.

• Cut the top off the squash, halve it, scoop out the seeds and chop into chunks. The skin is edible but you can peel it if you prefer.

• Place the squash in a roasting tin and give it a massage with some olive oil and seasoning. Spread into a single layer and roast for 30-40 minutes, or until the flesh is tender and the skin (if left on) is soft. Unpeeled squash will take slightly longer to cook but holds its shape better.

• Meanwhile, make the pesto. Place the basil leaves, crushed garlic, pine nuts, lemon juice and Parmesan into a food processor and pulse.

• Add the olive oil a little at a time until it forms a paste.

• Season with salt.
(Alternatively, grind all the ingredients except the oil with a pestle and mortar, then trickle in the oil).

• When the squash is cooked, lightly crush the hazelnuts and sprinkle on top. Drizzle with the pesto and serve with salad and couscous. Any pesto you don't use can be stored in a jar in the fridge.

Pumpkin and chickpea stew

A deliciously warming, cheap and easy family meal, that's packed with nutrients.

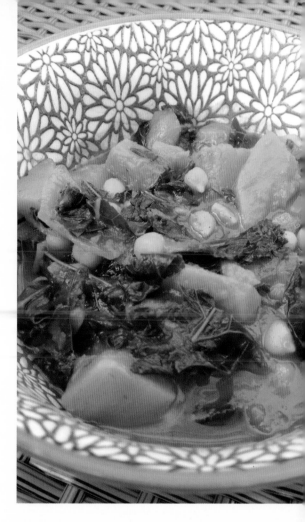

Serves 4-6
- **3 tablespoons sunflower oil**
- **2 onions, chopped**
- **4 cloves of garlic, chopped**
- **3cm piece of fresh ginger, finely chopped**
  (or ½ teaspoon ground ginger)
- **½ teaspoon ground cinnamon**
- **1 teaspoon ground turmeric**
- **1 teaspoon paprika**
- **400g tin of chickpeas, drained and rinsed**
- **900g pumpkin or squash, peeled and cut into chunks**
- **500g passata**
- **200g kale, chopped without stalks**
- **450ml vegetable stock**
- **Handful of coriander, chopped**

Method

- Heat the oil and saute the onions over a medium heat until soft.

- Turn the heat down slightly and add the garlic, ginger, dried spices and pumpkin or squash. Cook for another couple of minutes.

- Add the chickpeas, passata and stock so that the pumpkin is covered (add more stock if necessary.)

- Bring to the boil, then lower the heat, cover and simmer for about 20 minutes.

- Throw in the kale and simmer uncovered for another 10 minutes, or until everything is cooked.

- Scatter the coriander on top and serve.

Strawberries
♥ Love them

Nothing conjures up the taste of summer quite like a home-grown strawberry. They are so delicious that the health benefits are just a bonus really. But as strawberries are super-high in antioxidants there is even more reason to over indulge.

These splendid berries contain an army of beneficial flavonoids – including ellagic acid, anthocyanin, quercetin and kaempferol – that can help stave off serious illnesses. Strawberries are also a good source of vitamin C, as well as B vitamins and manganese which is important for numerous processes throughout the body.

Eating lots of strawberries as part of a balanced diet could contribute to a reduced risk of heart disease. This is because compounds in the berries have been shown to lower cholesterol levels by reducing the amount of LDL (bad) cholesterol in the blood.[49] Other studies have investigated the potential of strawberries to help protect the body against various types of cancer including oral, breast, colon and prostate.

And despite their wonderfully sweet flavour, strawberries contain much less sugar than many other fruits. In case this sounds too good to be true, 100g of strawberries has a total sugar content of 6.1 grams, compared to an average of 11.6 grams for apples, 16.1 grams for grapes, and 18.1 grams for bananas.[16] Eating strawberries after a meal may help to regulate blood sugar, reducing spikes in both glucose and insulin. This suggests they could offer some natural defence against type 2 diabetes.

Despite their glowing health benefits, shop-bought strawberries are one of the worst offenders when it comes to pesticides. According to the European Food Safety Authority (EFSA) strawberries are more likely to exceed legal limits for pesticide residues than any other fruit, and even organic ones may contain some traces of chemicals, which is perhaps an even more compelling reason to grow your own.

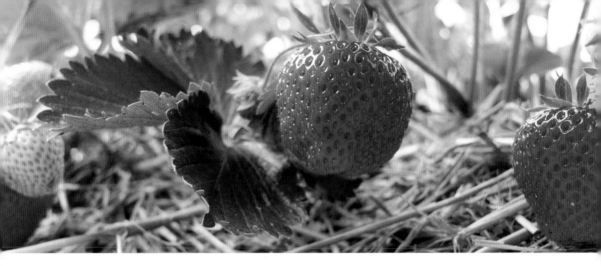

❀ Grow them

Gloriously summery and impossibly sweet, strawberries are a highlight of any kitchen garden or allotment. Shop-bought ones literally pale into insignificance in comparison. You don't even need a garden; strawberries are perfect for pots, hanging baskets and grow-bags, just as long as they have a sunny spot. In fact, growing strawberries this way can make them less of a target for slugs and other thieves.

When and how to plant

Strawberries are rarely grown from seed, and are usually bought as plants or bare-root runners (young plantlets.) These can be planted during spring, or between July and October, as long as the ground isn't too cold or wet.

Mail-order and online nurseries also sell cold-stored runners which have been kept at just below freezing point. These can be planted between March and July and should produce fruit within 60 days.

Before planting strawberries into the ground, remove any weeds and dig in some organic matter, like well-rotted manure, or garden compost, to enrich the soil.

Dig a small hole and insert the plant so that the roots are all underground, but the crown (the growing tip of the plant) is above soil level so it doesn't rot. Press the soil down around the plant so it's nice and firm. Leave gaps of about 35cm between each plant and 75cm between rows.

Water regularly at the base of the plant, avoiding the fruit and leaves. Once the flowers appear, feed once a week with a high-potassium feed like comfrey tea, as for tomatoes. Though if you don't manage to do this, don't despair – they will still taste nice!

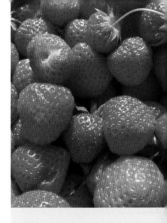

When the strawberries develop, place some straw, or other dry material, underneath them to keep them above the soil and prevent them from rotting. Another method is to grow the plants through polythene.

Resist picking the strawberries until they are completely red, as they won't ripen any further once picked.

After harvesting

Once the fruit has come to an end, remove the straw and cut back the old leaves, to encourage strong growth the following year.

Strawberry plants will carry on fruiting for about six years, but will become less productive after about four years, so it's a good idea to replace them. The easiest way to do this is to use the runners sent out by existing plants – these are the long stems that run across the ground and sprout baby plants. Simply peg them down with small hoops of bent wire, or hair grips. Although if you don't get round to it, they often just root themselves without intervention.

Once the new plant is well rooted (after about four weeks) snip the runner to separate it from the parent plant, then replant the baby in a new spot, or just leave it to grow where it is.

For best results, remove the flowers of new plants in the first season to encourage them to crop well in subsequent years. This is easier once you have an established patch of strawberries with some that are already in their prime.

Problems and troubleshooting

Slugs, snails, woodlice and birds all have an unwelcome passion for strawberries. Cover plants with netting to keep the birds away, and use straw to help deter slugs and snails. (See the section on salad for other ways of controlling slugs.)

Types of strawberry plants

There are two main categories of strawberry plants:

Summer-fruiting strawberries: these produce one big crop per year, over a two or three week period. There are early, mid and late season cultivars, so if you have enough space, grow some of each to extend the picking season.

Perpetual strawberries: also known as everbearing, these will keep producing smaller amounts of fruit from early summer until the autumn.

Varieties to try:

'Honeoye' – a prolific fruiter with firm, tasty berries. Early season.

'Elsanta' – one of the most popular and commonly grown varieties. Produces lots of large fruit with excellent flavour. Mid season.

'Florence'- large, glossy fruits with good flavour and disease resistance. Late season.

'Mara de Bois' – a perpetual variety with aromatic fruits that taste a bit like wild strawberries.

'Gariguette' – an old-fashioned gourmet French variety with elongated fruits, prized for their outstanding scent and flavour. Less prolific than modern varieties. An early cropper.

☺ Eat them

NO RECIPE CAN ever improve upon the taste of a perfectly-ripe, sun-warmed strawberry, or capture that just-picked sensation. But the following fusion of cultures and flavours comes a fairly close second.

Spanish almond cake with British strawberries

This cake recipe is an old Spanish hand-me-down, which just happens to sit beautifully with a pile of British strawberries. Modern versions of this almond cake call for the eggs to be separated with the whites whisked and folded in at the end, which gives a lighter texture. But there is something irresistibly dense and unrefined about the old-fashioned way. This is one of those occasions where sugar gets a reprieve.

- **200g ground almonds**
- **200g caster sugar**
- **4 eggs** (whole)
- **Zest of 1 lemon**
- **¼ teaspoon cinnamon**

For the strawberries
- **300g fresh strawberries**
- **Juice of 1 lemon**
- **2 tablespoons sugar**

Method

• Hull the strawberries and chop into quarters. Place in a bowl with the lemon juice and sugar and mix well. Cover and leave to stand for an hour or so, stirring occasionally.

For the cake

• Preheat the oven to 180°C/160°C fan/gas mark 4. Grease a 23cm cake tin with butter and dust with flour.

• Beat all the ingredients together and pour into the tin. And that's it!

• Cook in the oven for 30 minutes, or until done.

• Leave to cool then pile the strawberries on top.

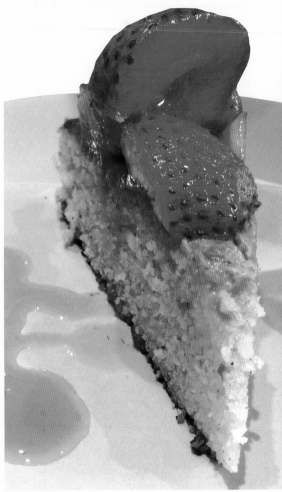

Dairy-free strawberry mousse cake

Deliciously light and creamy, this summery dessert is great for vegans and non-vegans alike. For an even easier option, just make the topping and serve it as a mousse.

Serves 10

Topping
- **2 tins of good quality, full fat coconut milk – placed in the fridge overnight**
- **300g strawberries plus extra to decorate**
- **2 tablespoons of honey**

Base
- **250g almonds**
- **200g dates, pitted**

Method

• The day before you make this put the unopened tins of coconut milk in the fridge.

• To make the base, soak the dates in hot water for 5 minutes, then drain completely.

• Put the almonds into a food processor and pulse until crumbly.

• Add the dates and pulse again until you get a sticky kind of dough.

• Grease a 22cm cake tin with coconut oil, and press the dough into the tin. Place in the freezer while you make the topping.

• Blend or mash the strawberries and honey. Don't worry about a few lumps.

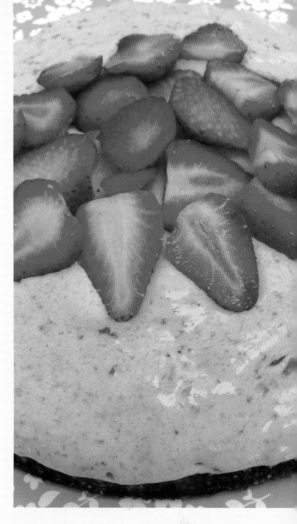

• Take the coconut milk out of the fridge, turn the tins upside down and open from the bottom, then pour off the watery bit (you can keep this to use in curries or smoothies). Whisk the remaining coconut solids until you have fluffy peaks.

• Fold the strawberries into the coconut cream, then pour the mixture over the base.

• Place in the freezer for an hour, then decorate with the remaining strawberries and serve. You can also leave it in the fridge to set, but it won't hold its shape quite as well.

Sweet potatoes

♥ Love them

The poor old potato has fallen from grace. These days it's all about the sweet potato, which is in fact no relation of the humble spud at all, not even a distant, twice-removed, remarried second cousin. Sweet potatoes are actually related to bindweed – but don't let that put you off – whereas ordinary potatoes belong to the tomato family.

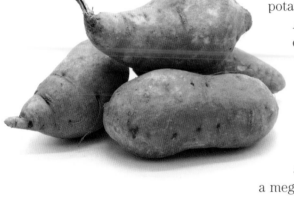

Although there is little difference in calories between sweet potatoes and regular potatoes, the sweet ones are much more nutritious and if boiled, rather than baked, they have a lower glycaemic index, so can help keep your blood sugar levels steady.

The orange-fleshed tubers (you can also get white and purple ones) provide a mega dose of vitamin A, in the form of beta-carotene. Just one serving of sweet potato, whether baked, steamed or raw, provides more than one hundred per cent of the RNI of vitamin A that is recommended daily. Sweet potatoes also contain vitamins B, C and E as well as antioxidants and minerals, especially potassium, magnesium, manganese and iron.

To get the full nutritional benefits of sweet potato, don't bother peeling them as the skins contain both fibre and nutrients. You can also eat the leaves which are one of the best kept 'superfood' secrets, being extremely nutritious and similar in taste to spinach. Never eat the leaves or stems of regular potatoes though as these are poisonous.

> You can also eat the leaves which are one of the best kept 'superfood' secrets, being extremely nutritious and similar in taste to spinach ...

❀ Grow them

There's no getting away from it; sweet potatoes are trickier to grow than your classic King Edwards or Maris Pipers. However, things are looking up as new hardier cultivars are now available.

Your chances of getting a decent crop are significantly improved if you have a greenhouse or polytunnel, as sweet potatoes need warm, humid conditions. But if not don't despair, it's still possible to grow these nutritional treasures in a garden or allotment. Just cover the soil with black plastic a month before planting to warm it up, and to increase your chances further still, cover the plants with cloches or fleece.

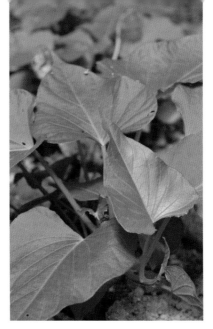

Planting

Sweet potatoes are usually grown from cuttings called 'slips'. These are best ordered online, to arrive at the end of April.

Sweet potato leaves growing above ground.

Before planting, place the slips in a glass of lukewarm water overnight, then plant them in pots the next day, making sure the stem is covered up to the lowest leaves. Keep the pots indoors.

Once the seedlings are about 10cm tall, harden them off to acclimatise them, then plant out in early June, in high ridges or mounds of fertile soil. Earthing up the soil in this way helps with drainage and warmth.

Plant seedlings at a depth of 5-8cm, leaving gaps of 25-30cm between plants. Keep plants well-watered, especially in the first few weeks. Sinking cut-off plastic bottles into the soil is a good way to get liquid down to the roots. Alternatively, sweet potatoes can be grown in large containers.

The foliage can grow at a fast and furious rate, so trim it back or train it up strings or a trellis if necessary – or pick the leaves to eat. Pinch out the growing points of stems once they reach 60cm, to encourage lateral growth.

Harvesting

Sweet potatoes are ready to harvest 12-16 weeks after planting, usually in October when the leaves turn yellow.

The longer the tubers stay in the ground the larger they will grow – but don't risk letting them encounter a frost, and take care not to damage them when digging them up.

Sweet potatoes will store for several months if they are 'cured' first. Do this by lying them in the sun for a week to toughen the skins.

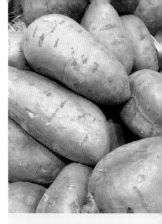

Varieties to try:

'Beauregard' – the most commonly grown variety in the UK with sweet orange flesh. Fast-maturing and reliable.

'Georgia Jet' – reliable and heavy cropping with purplish skin and orange flesh.

'O Henry' – bushier than other varieties and the cream-coloured tubers develop in clusters under the plant so are easier to harvest.

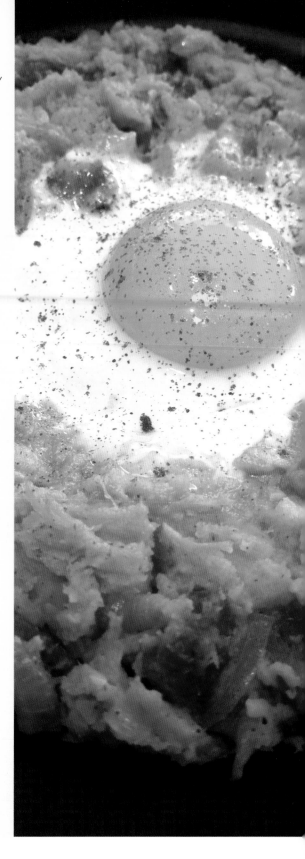

👄 Eat them

FIRST THERE WAS cauliflower rice, then came courgetti pasta, followed by kale crisps. And now: sweet potato toast. But the fact you can put a vegetable in a toaster, doesn't mean you should – unless of course you have actually run out of bread. Although even then, it's questionable.

One of my favourite, and laziest, ways to eat sweet potatoes is to hack them into wedges, season with paprika, and roast in the oven with some whole cloves of garlic, for around 40 minutes, although roasting sweet potatoes does bump up the GI, if that's something you're trying to avoid.

Fiery sweet potato hash and eggs

This heavenly hash can be whipped up for supper or a weekend breakfast in less than half an hour. The chorizo and chilli really kicks through the sweetness of the potato. Amazing!

Serves 4
- 3 or 4 sweet potatoes, peeled and diced
- 150g chorizo, chopped into cubes
- ½ green chilli, chopped
- 2 red onions, chopped
- 4 cloves garlic, chopped
- 4 eggs
- Sprinkling of paprika and black pepper

Method

- Plunge the diced sweet potatoes into a pan of salted water and bring to the boil. Simmer for a couple of minutes until half cooked, then drain and mash with a fork to break them up a bit.

- Heat up a frying pan and dry fry the chorizo for a few minutes until the oil is released.

- Remove the chorizo with a slotted spoon and set aside, leaving the oil in the pan.

- Add the onion and chilli to the pan and fry in the chorizo oil for a few minutes until soft. Add the garlic and cook for a couple more minutes.

- Return the chorizo to the pan, add the sweet potatoes and cook on a medium-high heat for 15- 20 minutes, turning from time to time and smashing the potato down with a spatula to flatten it. Add some oil if it gets too dry.

- When the sweet potato is starting to turn crispy at the edges, make four wells in the mixture, so that you can see the pan at the bottom. Crack one egg into each well and cook for a few minutes until the whites are done but the yolks are slightly runny.

- Sprinkle the paprika and pepper over the top and serve immediately.

Sweet potato, chicken and peanut butter curry

Don't be put off by the addition of peanut butter (unless the mere mention of it brings you out in hives); it gives a lovely rich consistency to this curry. For a veggie option, just replace the chicken with chickpeas. This makes plenty, but it freezes beautifully.

Serves 8
- 3 tablespoons sunflower oil
- 2 onions, sliced
- 1 fresh red chilli, finely chopped (optional)
- 5 cloves of garlic, crushed
- 4cm piece of fresh ginger, finely chopped
- 1 teaspoon ground coriander
- 1 teaspoon cayenne pepper
- 1 teaspoon ground cumin
- 700g sweet potatoes, peeled and roughly chopped
- 600g chicken breast or thighs, chopped into bite sized pieces
- 2 x 400g tins chopped tomatoes
- 2 large handfuls of spinach
- 500ml chicken or vegetable stock
- 150g peanut butter
- Handful of fresh coriander to finish

---•▸

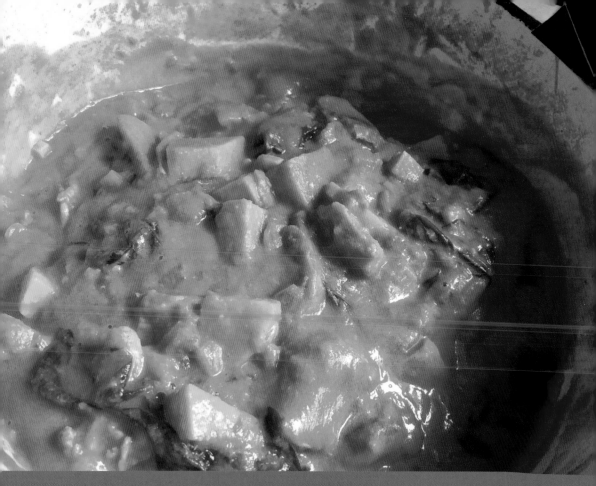

Method

• Heat the oil in a wok or deep frying pan and fry the onion for a few minutes until soft. Add the garlic, ginger, chilli and dried spices and cook for another couple of minutes.

• Add the sweet potato, chicken (or chickpeas) stock and tomatoes, so that everything is just covered – add extra stock if necessary.

• Bring to the boil, then reduce the heat and simmer for around 20 minutes or until the sweet potatoes are tender and the chicken is cooked.

• Stir in the peanut butter until the sauce becomes thick. Throw in the spinach and cook for a couple of minutes until wilted. Sprinkle the coriander on top and serve with rice.

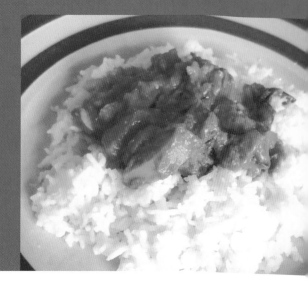

Tomatoes

♥ Love them

Tomatoes are one of the easiest ways to bump up your five, or ten, a day, as they feature in so many dishes. From pasta sauces to pizza, soups, curries, salads, even ketchup and cocktails, it's almost harder to avoid tomatoes, than it is to eat them, which is for most people rather fortunate, since they are a valuable source of vitamins A, C and E, as well as potassium. But the real super power of this family staple resides in the high concentration of lycopene, a potent antioxidant. Lycopene is the pigment that makes tomatoes red and although it's present in a few other fruits like watermelon, pink grapefruit and papaya, the vast majority of our intake in the West comes from tomatoes – the redder, the better.

Lycopene is part of the carotenoid family and is thought to be one of the most powerful antioxidants. Consequently, there has been much excitement about the role of tomatoes in protecting against chronic illnesses, including cancer. In particular, a number of studies have found that men who eat a diet rich in tomatoes or tomato-based products have a reduced risk of prostate cancer.[50] And it's thought that lycopene may offer protection against other forms of cancers too.

In addition, lycopene is thought to provide ammunition against cardiovascular disease by reducing LDL (bad) cholesterol and lowering blood pressure.[51] It can also help to keep skin looking young and healthy, by providing protection against UV damage.

Unlike most fruits and vegetables, the nutritional value of tomatoes is improved by cooking, as this makes the lycopene more bioavailable, or easily absorbed by the body. And as lycopene is fat soluble, don't hold back on the olive oil. Cooking does reduce the vitamin C content though, so it's good to eat both cooked and fresh tomatoes – not least for that unbeatable home-grown taste.

> Unlike most fruits and vegetables, the nutritional value of tomatoes is improved by cooking ...

❋ Grow them

Although fairly easy to grow, tomatoes are a crop that give as good as they get. If all you do is water them, you will probably end up with something edible. But for flavour that surpasses anything you can buy in a shop it's worth indulging them a little.

The type of seed, location, and unfortunately the weather, all help determine success or failure. If you have a greenhouse you can bypass the vagaries of the last one, otherwise it's essential to choose varieties that are suitable for outdoor growing.

Tomatoes fall into two main categories:

Bush (or determinate) varieties. These stop growing when they reach a specific height. Bush tomatoes are the easiest to grow because they don't need pruning and can often be grown in large pots or hanging baskets.

Cordon (or indeterminate) varieties, also known as vine tomatoes. These are grown as a single, tall stem and will need support and regular removal of side shoots.

How to grow tomatoes from seed

Around mid-March, sow seeds indoors in pots and cover with a sprinkling of potting compost. Water gently and keep damp. Plants destined for the greenhouse can be started off in February.

Place the pots inside a polythene bag or propagator to conserve

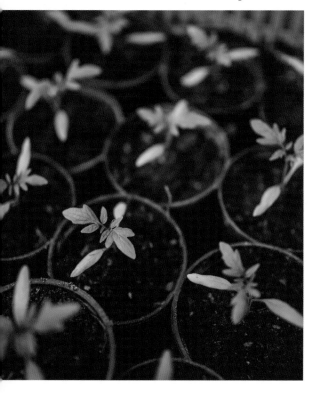

heat and moisture, or cover with clingfilm and leave in a sunny spot to grow. Remove covers once the seedlings emerge.

When the seedlings have a few leaves replant them into larger pots (you may need to do this a couple of times.)

In May or June (depending on the weather and where you live) bring the pots outside for a few hours each day to harden them off, remembering to take them in again at night. Do this for 7-10 days.

Once all chance of frost has passed, transplant your tomato plants to their final growing position outside. Choose a sunny, sheltered spot and mix some organic manure or compost into the soil. Allow 45cm between plants. Support cordon varieties by loosely tying the stems to a cane.

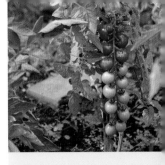

Growing care

For cordon varieties, snap off the side shoots as they appear. These are the shoots that grow between the stem and the main leaves. Once five or six trusses (branches) of fruit have formed cut off the top of the plant so the energy goes to the fruit. Bush varieties don't need pruning.

Feeding and watering

Water plants little and often. Irregular watering can cause the fruits to split or develop blossom end rot – unsightly black patches, due to calcium-deficiency from a lack of water.

Tomatoes are potassium-hungry plants and need feeding once a week once the flowers have appeared. Commercial fertilisers are available but you can easily make your own organic liquid feeds like comfrey tea (see the earlier section on super soil.)

Tips for success

When planting your tomatoes into the ground, sink a plastic bottle into the soil with both ends cut off. This provides a funnel through which you can water the deeper roots, though if this sounds a bit excessive, don't worry, it's not essential.

If your seedlings are a bit 'leggy' or lanky when you come to transplant them, simply plant them deeper into the ground, burying the lower leaves if necessary. This will help the plant to stand up and encourage new roots to form.

At the end of the summer, bring any green tomatoes indoors and place them on some newspaper with a banana to encourage them to ripen. Any that refuse to change colour can be turned into chutney.

Problems and troubleshooting

Blight – this is a fungal disease that causes fruit to turn brown and rot, especially during wet summers. Remove any fruit that show signs of the disease and avoid growing tomatoes in the same spot in consecutive years. Some varieties have been developed to be blight-resistant.

Whitefly – these tiny pests feed on tomato leaves and weaken the plant. Plant other strong smelling plants in the same area, such as nasturtiums, marigolds, or basil, as a repellent.

Varieties to try:

'Gardener's Delight' – produces bags of delicious, flavour-packed cherry tomatoes, usually grown as a cordon. A must-try.

'Tornado' – produces heavy crops of small, bright red fruit and is particularly suited to growing outdoors, even in cooler, wet climates. Ideal for hanging baskets or pots. A bush variety.

'Sweet Million' – produces long trusses of extremely sweet, cherry-sized fruits. Suitable for greenhouses, outdoors, or containers. A cordon variety.

'Ferline' – a beefsteak tomato with well-flavoured fruits that are resistant to blight. A cordon variety.

'Red Alert' – a popular, early maturing bush tomato, ideal for growing outdoors, or in containers.

👄 Eat them

Super BLT salad with garlic croutons and a yoghurt dressing

The favourite sarnie gets a makeover with more salad, less bread and a healthy dressing.

Serves 4
- **160g smoked bacon lardons or pancetta cubes**
- **1 Romaine lettuce, chopped**
- **Plenty of tomatoes, halved or chopped, depending on size**
- **1 cucumber, chopped**
- **1 avocado, cut into chunks**
- **Handful of black olives, halved**

For the croutons
- **A loaf, or part loaf, of stale bread. Seeded is good, but anything you have is fine**
- **20g butter**
- **20ml of olive oil**
- **3 garlic cloves, crushed**
- **1 tablespoon of fresh parsley, finely chopped**
- **Salt and pepper to season**

For the dressing
- **100ml natural yoghurt**
- **1 tablespoon white wine vinegar**
- **1 tablespoon lemon juice**
- **2 teaspoons wholegrain mustard**
- **1 teaspoon runny honey**
- **1 tablespoon olive oil**
- **Salt and pepper to season**

Method

- Preheat the oven to 180°C/160°C fan/gas 4.

- To make the croutons, tear the bread into small pieces, or chop into cubes, and place in a large bowl.

- Melt the butter in a saucepan with the olive oil. Stir in the garlic and parsley and season with salt and pepper.

- Drizzle the melted butter mixture over the bread so the pieces are evenly coated.

- Spread the bread in a single layer on a baking tray and bake until golden brown and crispy. This can take anything from 5 – 15 minutes, depending on the type and age of bread. The older the bread, the more quickly it will cook, so keep an eye on it! If you have more croutons than you need, they will keep for a few days in an airtight container or bag.

For the dressing
- Whisk all the ingredients together, or place them in a jam jar with the lid tightly closed and give it an energetic shake.

For the salad
- Fry the lardons or pancetta until crispy. Allow to cool slightly.

- Chop the lettuce, tomatoes and cucumber and combine in a bowl. Mix in the avocado and olives, then add the pancetta.

- Scatter the croutons on top, drizzle with the dressing and enjoy.

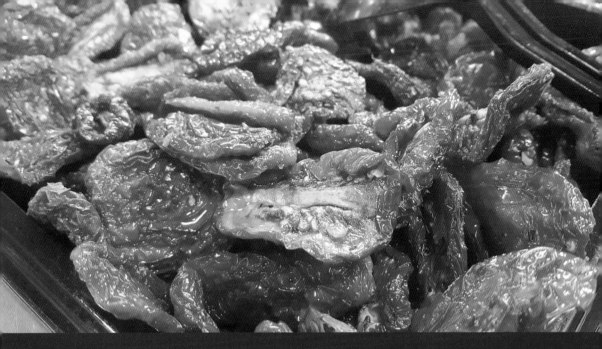

Slow-roasted tomatoes

The jars of 'sun-dried' tomatoes found in shops are often oily, chewy and expensive. But it's easy to make your own improved version, especially if you have a glut of tomatoes. Don't rely on the sun for roasting though – an oven comes in handy here. Unless of course you live in the south of Italy.

- **1kg tomatoes**
- **3 tablespoons olive oil, plus more if you plan to store the tomatoes**
- **2 sprigs of fresh thyme, broken up**
- **1 tablespoon fresh oregano, chopped** (or 1 teaspoon dried oregano)
- **1 teaspoon caster sugar**
- **5 cloves of garlic, peeled and roughly sliced**
- **Salt and pepper to season**

Method

- Preheat the oven to 100°C/gas 4.

- Cut the tomatoes into quarters, or halves if they are very small.

- Place the tomatoes in a shallow roasting tin, with the cut side facing up. Drizzle with the olive oil and scatter over the thyme, oregano, garlic and sugar. Season with salt and pepper.

- Cook the tomatoes for around 4 hours until the skins are wrinkly and the flesh has dried out. They may need longer, depending on the size of the tomatoes and how dry you want them to be. You can remove any smaller ones that cook faster than the rest.

- The tomatoes are delicious eaten straight away; in sandwiches, pasta, salads or just on their own. Or you can store them in a jar topped up with olive oil. They will keep for about a week in the fridge this way.

Watercress

♥ Love it

Although a relative newcomer on the superfood block, the Victorians couldn't get enough of this peppery green. Back in the nineteenth century, it was eaten by rich and poor, young and old. And we're talking handfuls, not just a token garnish on the edge of the plate.

By today's standards, the life of the average Victorian was positively gruelling; devoid of our own comforts and conveniences, and lacking in modern medicine.

Yet research suggests they were an astonishingly healthy bunch. According to an extensive examination of medical records, the Victorians were 90 per cent less likely to develop cancer, dementia and coronary artery disease than we are today. Meanwhile, obesity and related conditions were almost unheard of, especially among the working classes.[52] This enviable track record in disease-dodging, seems to be strongly correlated with a highly nutritious diet, involving around ten portions of seasonal fruit and veg a day, including copious quantities of watercress, which was cheap and abundantly available.

Watercress is no longer so economical – especially since being rebranded as a superfood. Yet it is packed with vitamins K, C, and A and is a great source of calcium, manganese and potassium. It also contains a number of B vitamins, vitamin E, magnesium, and phosphorus. What's more, the mustardy-tasting leaves contain high levels of organic compounds called glucosinolates. These are transformed into powerful molecules called isothiocyanates and there is evidence that these may inhibit various types of cancer.[53, 54]

And finally, in an analysis of 'powerhouse fruit and vegetables' which rated food for their nutrient density, watercress was given the highest score out of a total of forty-seven fruits and vegetables[55]

it is packed with vitamins K, C, and A and is a great source of calcium, manganese and potassium ...

leading some to claim that watercress really is the king, or queen, of superfoods.

The Victorians might have laughed at such a notion, but it seems we could do a lot worse than follow in our great-great-great-grandparents' dietary footsteps.

❀ Grow it

If you have always assumed you need a babbling brook running through your back garden to grow your own watercress, then you will be pleased to know you don't. If you do happen to have a private stream at your disposal, then great. If not, it will grow perfectly well in containers, window boxes, or in the ground.

Watercress can be grown from seed, which is sold in garden centres or online. Or you can buy fresh watercress and take some cuttings.

For cuttings, it's best to use bunched watercress, rather than the bagged stuff. Simply take some stems and immerse them in a jar of water until they form roots. Change the water if it becomes a bit murky. Once your stems are well-rooted plant them in some wet soil.

Or to grow from scratch, sprinkle some seed onto the surface of damp soil. Don't cover with compost, but leave on a windowsill to grow. Empty fruit punnets with holes in the bottom make excellent containers, sat inside a dish of water to keep the soil soaked.

Watercress can be grown indoors at any time of the year as it doesn't need much heat to germinate, so it's perfect for growing in the kitchen for a ready-to-eat supply.

For outdoors, it's best to wait until March before sowing. Watercress thrives in containers or you can sow it straight into the ground. All you need to do then is keep the soil moist – this is one crop where you don't need to worry about over-watering. Placing the pot inside a larger shallow container or tray means it's less likely to dry out. Just remember to top it up with water now and then.

In early summer, you could give your watercress an extra boost with some nettle tea.

Baby watercress will be ready to eat after about 21 days. For larger leaves, leave it another week or so. Snip the shoots just above ground level and they will happily grow back again.

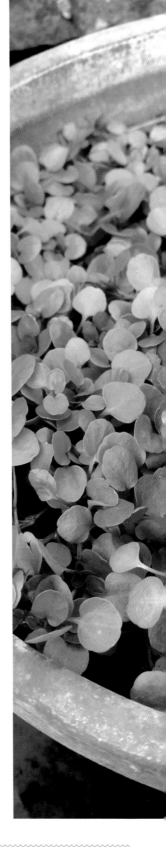

ᕦ🫦ᕤ Eat it

THE VICTORIANS ATE watercress stuffed between pieces of bread, or rolled up like an ice cream cone. Not quite a Mr Whippy, but definitely more nutritious. It gives a peppery kick to salads, soup, potatoes and omelettes, or you can sauté it with olive oil until the leaves are wilted and slightly crispy. It also goes particularly well with fish.

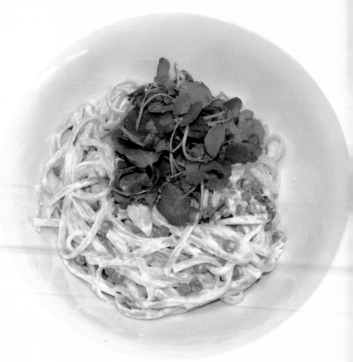

Linguine with salmon and watercress

Blissfully quick and easy, this makes a perfect mid-week meal.

Serves 4
- **400g linguine**
- **2 salmon fillets**
- **200ml tub crème fraîche**
- **Zest of ½ lemon and a squeeze of juice**
- **200g peas**
- **100g watercress, roughly chopped plus a little extra to garnish**

Method

• Place the salmon in a pan, skin side up and cover with cold water. Bring to the boil then simmer for 5 minutes or until cooked. Alternatively, cook under a grill. Remove the skin, then flake the flesh and set aside.

• Cook the pasta for 10 minutes, or according to the packet instructions, adding the peas for the last few minutes.

• Meanwhile, place the crème fraîche in a saucepan, add the lemon and simmer for 5 minutes.

• Season to taste with salt and pepper.

• Drain the pasta and peas and stir in the watercress, salmon and crème fraîche.

• Garnish with extra watercress.

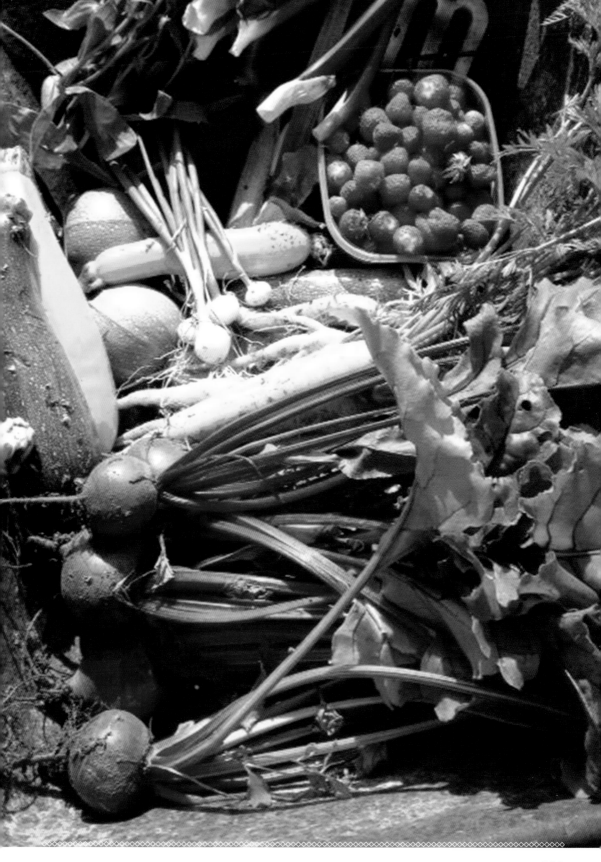

Endnotes

1. Barański M, Średnicka-Tober D, Volakakis N, et al. Higher antioxidant and lower cadmium concentrations and lower incidence of pesticide residues in organically grown crops: a systematic literature review and meta-analyses. *The British Journal of Nutrition.*

2. https://www.gov.uk/government/collections/pesticide-residues-in-food-results-of-monitoring-programme

3. https://www.gov.uk/government/uploads/system/uploads/attachment_data/file/540705/pesticide-residues-2015-crop-sector-berries.pdf

4. Regulation (EC) No 1924/2006 which came in to effect July 2007

5. 2014;112(5):794-811. doi:10.1017/S0007114514001366.2. Pittler MH, White AR, Stevinson C, Ernst E. Effectiveness of artichoke extract in preventing alcohol-induced hangovers: a randomized controlled trial. *CMAJ: Canadian Medical Association Journal.* 2003;169(12):1269-1273.

6. Carlsen MH, Halvorsen BL, Holte K, et al. The total antioxidant content of more than 3100 foods, beverages, spices, herbs and supplements used worldwide. *Nutrition Journal.* 2010;9:3. doi:10.1186/1475-2891-9-3.

7. Rondanelli M, Giacosa A, Morazzoni P, et al. MediterrAsian Diet Products That Could Raise HDL-Cholesterol: A Systematic Review. *BioMed Research International.* 2016;2016:2025687. doi:10.1155/2016/2025687.

8. Englisch W, Beckers C, Unkauf M, Ruepp M, Zinserling V. Efficacy of artichoke dry extract in patients with hyperlipoproteinemia. Arzneimittel-Forschung. 2000;50(3):260–5. PUBMED: 10758778

9. Mileo AM, Di Venere D, Abbruzzese C, Miccadei S. Long Term Exposure to Polyphenols of Artichoke (Cynara scolymus L.) Exerts Induction of Senescence Driven Growth Arrest in the MDA-MB231 Human Breast Cancer Cell Line. *Oxidative Medicine and Cellular Longevity.* 2015;2015:363827. doi:10.1155/2015/363827.

10. Pulito C, Mori F, Sacconi A, et al. *Cynara scolymus* affects malignant pleural mesothelioma by promoting apoptosis and restraining invasion. *Oncotarget.* 2015;6(20):18134-18150.

11. Clifford T, Howatson G, West DJ, Stevenson EJ. The Potential Benefits of Red Beetroot Supplementation in Health and Disease. *Nutrients.* 2015;7(4):2801-2822. doi:10.3390/nu7042801.

12. Siervo M., Lara J., Ogbonmwan I., Mathers J.C. Inorganic nitrate and beetroot juice supplementation reduces blood pressure in adults: a systematic review and meta-analysis. J. Nutr. 2013;143:818–826.

13. Govind J. Kapadia, Magnus A. Azuine, G. Subba Rao, Takanari Arai, Akira Iida, Harukuni Tokuda. Cytotoxic Effect of the Red Beetroot (Beta vulgaris L.) Extract Compared to Doxorubicin (Adriamycin) in the Human Prostate (PC-3) and Breast (MCF-7) Cancer Cell Lines. 2011. Anti-Cancer Agents in Medicinal Chemistry. Volume 11, issue 3, Eureka Science Ltd. 280-284.

14. Presley TD, Morgan AR, Bechtold E, et al. Acute effect of a high nitrate diet on brain perfusion in older adults. *Nitric oxide : biology and chemistry / official journal of the Nitric Oxide Society.* 2011;24(1):34-42. doi:10.1016/j.niox.2010.10.002.

15. Jones AM. Dietary Nitrate Supplementation and Exercise Performance. *Sports Medicine (Auckland, N.z)*. 2014;44(Suppl 1):35-45. doi:10.1007/s40279-014-0149-y.

16. McCance & Widdowson, The Composition of Foods, 5th Ed, RSC & MAFF

17. Diaconeasa, Z.; Leopold, L.; Rugină, D.; Ayvaz, H.; Socaciu, C. Antiproliferative and Antioxidant Properties of Anthocyanin Rich Extracts from Blueberry and Blackcurrant Juice. *Int. J. Mol. Sci. 2015, 16,* 2352-2365

18. Fung TT, Chiuve SE, Willett WC, Hankinson SE, Hu FB, Holmes MD. Intake of specific fruits and vegetables in relation to risk of estrogen receptor-negative breast cancer among postmenopausal women. *Breast cancer research and treatment.* 2013;138(3):925-930. doi:10.1007/s10549-013-2484-3.

19. Hurst, S. M., McGhie, T. K., Cooney, J. M., Jensen, D. J., Gould, E. M., Lyall, K. A. and Hurst, R. D. (2010), Blackcurrant proanthocyanidins augment IFN-γ-induced suppression of IL-4 stimulated CCL26 secretion in alveolar epithelial cells. Mol. Nutr. Food Res., 54: S159–S170. doi:10.1002/mnfr.200900297

20. Cassidy A, Franz M, Rimm EB. Dietary flavonoid intake and incidence of erectile dysfunction. *The American Journal of Clinical Nutrition.* 2016;103(2):534-541. doi:10.3945/ajcn.115.122010.

21. Cassidy A, Mukamal KJ, Liu L, Franz M, Eliassen AH, Rimm EB. A high anthocyanin intake is associated with a reduced risk of myocardial infarction in young and middle-aged women. *Circulation.* 2013;127(2):188-196. doi:10.1161/CIRCULATIONAHA.112.122408.

22. Whyte AR & Williams CM (2015). A pilot study investigating the effects of a single dose of a flavonoid-rich blueberry drink on memory in 8-10 year old children. Nutrition, 31: 531-534

23. Mehran S.M. M, B. G. Simultaneous Determination of Levodopa and Carbidopa from Fava Bean, Green Peas and Green Beans by High Performance Liquid Gas Chromatography. *Journal of Clinical and Diagnostic Research* : JCDR. 2013;7(6):1004-1007. doi:10.7860/JCDR/2013/5415.3072.

24. Armah CN, Derdemezis C, Traka MH, et al. Diet rich in high glucoraphanin broccoli reduces plasma LDL cholesterol: Evidence from randomised controlled trials. *Molecular Nutrition & Food Research.* 2015;59(5):918-926. doi:10.1002/mnfr.201400863.

25. Tortorella, Stephanie M. et al. "Dietary Sulforaphane in Cancer Chemoprevention: The Role of Epigenetic Regulation and HDAC Inhibition." *Antioxidants & Redox Signaling* 22.16 (2015): 1382–1424. PMC. Web. 21 June 2017.

26. Singh K, Connors SL, Macklin EA, et al. Sulforaphane treatment of autism spectrum disorder (ASD). *Proceedings of the National Academy of Sciences of the United States of America.* 2014;111(43):15550-15555. doi:10.1073/pnas.1416940111.

27. Victoria A. Kirsh et al. Prospective Study of Fruit and Vegetable Intake and Risk of Prostate Cancer. Journal of the National Cancer Institute (2007) 99 (15): 1200-1209. Published by Oxford University Press.

28. Chaurasia S et al. Biochemical Studies on Antioxidant Potential of Green Beans in Fresh and Processed Conditions. American Journal of PharmTech Research 2012.

29. Maria Neve Ombra, Antonio d'Acierno, Filomena Nazzaro, et al., "Phenolic Composition and Antioxidant and Antiproliferative Activities of the Extracts of Twelve

Common Bean (Phaseolus vulgaris L.) Endemic Ecotypes of Southern Italy before and after Cooking," Oxidative Medicine and Cellular Longevity, vol. 2016, Article ID 1398298, 12 pages, 2016. doi:10.1155/2016/1398298

30. Mirabi P, Alamolhoda SH, Esmaeilzadeh S, Mojab F. Effect of Medicinal Herbs on Primary Dysmenorrhoea- a Systematic Review . *Iranian Journal of Pharmaceutical Research* : IJPR. 2014;13(3):757-767.

31. Delaram M, Kheiri S, Hodjati MR. Comparing the Effects of Echinophora-platyloba, Fennel and Placebo on Pre-menstrual Syndrome. *Journal of Reproduction & Infertility.* 2011;12(3):221-226.

32. Alexandrovich I, Rakovitskaya O, Kolmo E, et al. The effect of fennel (Foeniculum vulgare) seed oil emulsion in infantile colic: a randomized, placebo-controlled study. *Altern Ther Health Med.* 2003;9:58-61.

33. Bradley JM, Organ CL, Lefer DJ. Garlic-Derived Organic Polysulfides and Myocardial Protection. *The Journal of Nutrition.* 2016;146(2):403S-409S. doi:10.3945/jn.114.208066.

34. Ried K, Fakler P. Potential of garlic (*Allium sativum*) in lowering high blood pressure: mechanisms of action and clinical relevance. *Integrated Blood Pressure Control.* 2014;7:71-82. doi:10.2147/IBPC.S51434.

35. Nicastro HL, Ross SA, Milner JA. Garlic and onions: Their cancer prevention properties. *Cancer prevention research (Philadelphia, Pa).* 2015;8(3):181-189. doi:10.1158/1940-6207.CAPR-14-0172.

36. Zardast M, Namakin K, Esmaelian Kaho J, Hashemi SS. Assessment of antibacterial effect of garlic in patients infected with *Helicobacter pylori* using urease breath test. *Avicenna Journal of Phytomedicine.* 2016;6(5):495-501.

37. Jin Z-Y, Wu M, Han R-Q, et al. Raw garlic consumption as a protective factor for lung cancer, a population-based case-control study in a Chinese population. Cancer prevention research (Philadelphia, Pa). 2013;6(7):711-718. doi:10.1158/1940-6207.CAPR-13-0015.

38. Chen AY, Chen YC. A review of the dietary flavonoid, kaempferol on human health and cancer chemoprevention. *Food chemistry.* 2013;138(4):2099-2107. doi:10.1016/j.foodchem.2012.11.139.

39. Park S, Sapkota K, Kim S, Kim H, Kim S. Kaempferol acts through mitogen-activated protein kinases and protein kinase B/AKT to elicit protection in a model of neuroinflammation in BV2 microglial cells. *British Journal of Pharmacology.* 2011;164(3):1008-1025. doi:10.1111/j.1476-5381.2011.01389.x.

40. Kong L, Luo C, Li X, Zhou Y, He H. The anti-inflammatory effect of kaempferol on early atherosclerosis in high cholesterol fed rabbits. *Lipids in Health and Disease.* 2013;12:115. doi:10.1186/1476-511X-12-115.

41. Nicastro HL, Ross SA, Milner JA. Garlic and onions: Their cancer prevention properties. *Cancer prevention research (Philadelphia, Pa).* 2015;8(3):181-189. doi:10.1158/1940-6207.CAPR-14-0172.

42. Brüll V, Burak C, Stoffel-Wagner B, et al. Effects of a quercetin-rich onion skin extract on 24 h ambulatory blood pressure and endothelial function in overweight-to-obese patients with (pre-)hypertension: a randomised double-blinded placebo-controlled cross-over trial. *The British Journal of Nutrition.* 2015;114(8):1263-1277. doi:10.1017/S0007114515002950.

43. Jung JY, Lim Y, Moon MS, Kim JY, Kwon O. Onion peel extracts ameliorate hyperglycemia and insulin resistance in high fat diet/streptozotocin-induced diabetic rats. *Nutrition & Metabolism*. 2011;8:18. doi:10.1186/1743-7075-8-18.

44. Young SN. Folate and depression—a neglected problem. *Journal of Psychiatry & Neuroscience*. 2007;32(2):80-82.

45. Bazzano LA, Thompson AM, Tees MT, Nguyen CH, Winham DM. Non-Soy Legume Consumption Lowers Cholesterol Levels: A Meta-Analysis of Randomized Controlled Trials. *Nutrition, metabolism, and cardiovascular diseases : NMCD*. 2011;21(2):94-103. doi:10.1016/j.numecd.2009.08.012.

46. Burton-Freeman BM, Sandhu AK, Edirisinghe I. Red Raspberries and Their Bioactive Polyphenols: Cardiometabolic and Neuronal Health Links. *Advances in Nutrition*. 2016;7(1):44-65. doi:10.3945/an.115.009639.

47. Wang L-S, Arnold M, Huang Y-W, et al. Modulation of Genetic and Epigenetic Biomarkers of Colorectal Cancer in Humans by Black Raspberries: A Phase I Pilot Study. *Clinical cancer research : an official journal of the American Association for Cancer Research*. 2011;17(3):598-610. doi:10.1158/1078-0432.CCR-10-1260.

48.Gomes MB, Negrato CA. Alpha-lipoic acid as a pleiotropic compound with potential therapeutic use in diabetes and other chronic diseases. *Diabetology & Metabolic Syndrome*. 2014;6:80. doi:10.1186/1758-5996-6-80.

49. José M. Alvarez-Suarez, Francesca Giampieri, Sara Tulipani, Tiziana Casoli, Giuseppina Di Stefano, Ana M. González-Paramás, Celestino Santos-Buelga, Franco Busco, Josè L. Quiles, Mario D. Cordero, Stefano Bompadre, Bruno Mezzetti, Maurizio Battino. "One-month strawberry-rich anthocyanin supplementation ameliorates cardiovascular risk, oxidative stress markers and platelet activation in humans". *Journal of Nutritional Biochemistry* 25 (3): 289–294, March 2014.

50. Zu K, Mucci L, Rosner BA, et al. Dietary Lycopene, Angiogenesis, and Prostate Cancer: A Prospective Study in the Prostate-Specific Antigen Era. *JNCI Journal of the National Cancer Institute*. 2014;106(2):djt430. doi:10.1093/jnci/djt430. Published by Oxford University Press

51. Arab L, Steck S. Lycopene and cardiovascular disease. *Am J Clin Nutr*. 2000;71:1691S-1695S.

52. Clayton P, Rowbotham J. How the Mid-Victorians Worked, Ate and Died. *International Journal of Environmental Research and Public Health*. 2009;6(3):1235-1253. doi:10.3390/ijerph6031235.

53. Syed Alwi SS, Cavell BE, Telang U, Morris ME, Parry BM, Packham G. In vivo modulation of 4E binding protein 1 (4E-BP1) phosphorylation by watercress: a pilot study. *The British journal of nutrition*. 2010;104(9):1288-1296. doi:10.1017/S0007114510002217.

54. Gupta P, Wright SE, Kim S-H, Srivastava SK. Phenethyl Isothiocyanate: A comprehensive review of anti-cancer mechanisms. *Biochimica et biophysica acta*. 2014;1846(2):405-424. doi:10.1016/j.bbcan.2014.08.003.

55. Di Noia J. Defining Powerhouse Fruits and Vegetables: A Nutrient Density Approach. *Preventing Chronic Disease*. 2014;11:E95. doi:10.5888/pcd11.130390.

Acknowledgements

With grateful thanks to everyone who helped out trying, testing and photographing recipes: Kate, James, Lucy, Ed, Lizzie, Rosie, Zoe, and of course, Jonas, Daisy, Anya and Uli.

Words and images: Becky Dickinson.

Additional photography courtesy of Pixabay.

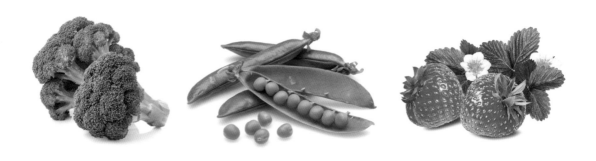

Notes

Notes

Notes

Notes